M000019585

The Tao of Teenagers

A Guide to Teen Health, Happiness & Empowerment

Peter Berg, Ed.D.

© 2016 by Peter Berg, Ed.D. All rights reserved.

No part of this book may be reproduced in any written, electronic, recording, or photocopying form without written permission of the author, Peter Berg, Ed.D., or the publisher, Youth Transformations Publishing.

Published by: Youth Transformations Publishing, Derry, New Hampshire
Cover Design by: Faye Designs
Editing by: Laurie Driggers

Books may be purchased in quantity and/or special sales by contacting the publisher, Youth Transformations Publishing, by email at peter@youthtransformations.com.

Printed in the United States of America

ISBN-13: 9780692756799

The Tao of Teenagers: A Guide to Teen Health, Happiness & Empowerment

Acknowledgements

This book is truly a collaboration between myself and the thousands of teenagers and adults I have had the pleasure to meet and work with. I am grateful for all the teens and adults courageous enough to be introspective and honestly share their experiences that have helped shape this book.

First and foremost, I want to dedicate this book to my soul mate, Laurie, whose help, support and encouragement was critical to the writing of this book and to my family and friends who have always been the source of my resolve. All of you are the foundation of who I am and the work that I am able to do.

I want to thank my coach, Kim Johnson, who pushed me forward through this process, and Jerry Mintz, the Executive Director of the Alternative Education Resource Organization, for his guidance.

I have been blessed with many wonderful teen and adult mentors, who, because of their inspiration, have made this book possible. To the teens that are brave enough to demand a healthy, happy, empowered life and the adults who want to help them get there, I thank you.

Table of Contents

Introduction

"Can I let it out?" "Yes, go ahead," I said, as I had this bright, strong, funny, emotional teenager in a safety hold. I felt his body go limp. What started as an attempt to hurt himself ended with an emotional and physical release and with a window into what he was going through. As he sobbed and talked about some of what he was dealing with and many aspects of his life, he said, "I just wanted to be happy."

Having had this experience so early in my work with teenagers shaped the many hours and years to come. It opened up a window for me into a big-picture, integrated view of health and happiness for teenagers. His story and the stories of the many teenagers I have worked with over the past 25 years have inspired me to write this book. I often think back to that moment and how it led me down a path of discovery and learning with and from teenagers, parents and caring adults.

Over the next 20-plus years, I came to know that health and happiness are inextricably linked. Indeed, it is difficult to separate these two states of being when looked at from a holistic, integrated view. You may notice that throughout this book I use the phrases 'health and happiness' and 'happiness and health' interchangeably; that's because the meaning is the same no matter the sequence.

Though I do not have children of my own, I have had the good fortune of working with teenagers in a variety of settings, from public and private schools, to therapeutic environments, including wilderness therapy, to a private coaching practice.

The teenage years, also referred to as adolescence — though in some discussions adolescence is viewed as anywhere from ages 12 to 24, in part, mostly due to the profound changes in the way the brain works during this time — is the most amazing and yet challenging time of our lives. Today's teenagers have many challenges that impact their health and happiness; in some respects, more than they ever have. In today's world, we have unprecedented access to information and ways of connecting with people and yet many teens report feeling disconnected, overwhelmed and anxious.

The National Institute of Mental Health estimates that 25% of teenagers deal with recurring anxiety that interferes with their daily lives and well-being. While a good number of teens feel they are technologically literate and are able to leverage it in a variety of ways, many still express feeling disconnected from each other and the world.

Teens are also bombarded with so many conflicting messages about what it means to be happy and healthy that it's no wonder they are confused and frustrated. The teens I have worked and continue to work with have repeatedly expressed their annoyance about the misconceptions some adults have about them and the way they are often portrayed in our culture. As one teen put it, "Because we're teenagers doesn't mean we don't care about our health. We sometimes do crazy things — eat junk food, stay up late and don't always listen to adults — but we care, even if it doesn't look like it."

The teenage years provide wonderful opportunities for exploration, self-discovery and growth. In essence, the teenage years are a time of immense opportunity. These years are often referred to as a time of great turmoil, and as sure as any teen knows or anyone who has spent time with teens knows, the amount of changes can be intense. This is precisely the time to seize this incredible opportunity to shape the path to lifelong health and happiness. While every person is an individual with unique needs and ways of being that need to be honored, I have found commonalities that, if in place, can help to pave the way for teens to be happy and healthy.

This book is part reflection, part research and part story sharing. It is important that we tell and share our stories. That is why this book contains the stories and reflections of the wonderful, brilliant, compassionate teenagers who I have had the pleasure to work with and continue to work with (of course, the situations have been changed so that any possible identifying information is omitted or altered beyond recognition). I also shared my personal stories and reflections where they seemed to fit. My own personal journey though my teenage years were, in part, very similar to that of other teenagers and in other ways unique to me.

All of the suggestions in this book have been tried, implemented and studied. This book is not about trying to get anyone — whether teen or adult — to do things 'my way'. It's truly about sharing experiences. Ultimately, it is you who will decide whether to dive deeper into what's in this book or to use it in any way.

How To Use This Book

Disclaimer. This book contains suggestions for teen health and happiness, and they are just that, suggestions. In no way should they be construed as medical advice or interventions. Treatment for any physical or mental condition should be conducted by your healthcare professional. I am not a physician, nor am I prescribing any medical treatments. Before implementing any suggestions or undertaking any new protocols, you should always consult with your healthcare professional.

Partnership/Empowerment. Whether you're a teen or adult, this book is best approached from a partnership mindset; partnership with yourself, with the information and suggestions in this book and partnership with teens and adults. This book is also about empowerment; if you're a teen, to know that you can take charge of your health and happiness, and if you're an adult, to know that you can be an instrumental partner in this empowerment.

Examples/Suggestions. There are real-life examples throughout this book. They are included with the hope that they can provide a starting point more than a how-to. They are also there for inspiration, to show that we are not alone and that many have shared our path at least in part. The suggestions that I have included at the end of most of the chapters are, again, just that, suggestions. The suggestions are based on the real-life experiences of the teenagers I have been blessed to have spent time with, and to a small degree, my own experiences.

Have Fun. Don't worry about trying to put every suggestion into practice at once. If you forget to do something or go outside of the suggestions, have fun with it. Have fun exploring and discovering new things.

Be Flexible/Use What Works. I hope you will find the suggestions and information in this book to be helpful and practical. I also hope that you remain flexible and use what you feel will work and what you can implement. If something works for you, great. If something doesn't work for you or doesn't resonate with you, then either put it aside for another time or ditch it. Be flexible and innovative. Make adjustments to the suggestions so that they work for you. There is no right or wrong way.

Read With An Open Mind And Heart. If you come across parts of this book that seem odd, too new-agey, hippy dippy, tree-huggerish or that don't fit for you, that's okay. I would invite you to consider why I would choose to include these things in a book like this.

This book is not about trying to convince anyone of anything. It's about sharing experiences. You may read particular parts and come away thinking, this guy is crazy. While that will come as no surprise to those who know me, I don't believe there is anything in this book that is so outrageous that it cannot be considered.

Not Comprehensive. The suggestions, reflections and focal points in this book are not meant to be a comprehensive plan for teen health and happiness. They are what I have found over the years to be the areas that get overlooked or are lacking when it comes to teen health and happiness. Or better yet, when given attention, these aspects can provide a path to teen health and happiness. As you will find as you read through this book, there are attributes that have not been addressed or discussed. This does not mean that they aren't important. It is more about leaving room for self-discovery.

For Dialogue. Use this whole book or parts of this book to generate dialogue. I have found that dialogue is more about an exploration of ideas and issues where people are committed to listening deeply to and learning from each other and putting aside their views, at least for the interim, as they search for true understanding. Discussion generally differs in that it's more about presenting opposing views and working to convince the other side to adopt that view or at least put practices in place that support that view.

Listen To Your Intuition. People like telling others what to do, and yes, I recommend following the advice of your medical professional. When it comes to this book, I hope that you listen to your intuition as well as considering the suggestions. You are the master.

Chapter One

What Is A Happy, Healthy Teen?

"So now you're going to tell me all the things I need to be happy and healthy?" "Yes and no," I said. "What do you mean?" My answer was that we were going to take an objective look at what was going on for this teen to see if there were any changes they wanted to make.

It's not about fitting into a certain criteria; if you have all these things, then you're happy and healthy, and if you don't, you're not. Plus, the truth is that happiness and health are ever-changing. It is unrealistic to think that any person is going to be completely happy all the time. In fact, feeling unhappy sometimes is natural and healthy, in that it means we can feel different emotions but also have a way to process them.

Being healthy is similar. There are many things we can do to maintain optimal health; however, there will be times when we are not in a state of optimal health for a variety of reasons. The key is to have ways to move back in the direction of optimal health and happiness.

Teenagers and adults have often asked me, why make the distinction between teenagers and adults? Don't teenagers and adults need the same things to be happy and healthy? Fundamentally, yes, there are aspects that are common to both teenage and adult health and happiness, yet there are differences in what an adult may need and what a teenager may need to be healthy and happy.

Let's take happiness, that often-elusive state of being that we all aspire to. What does it mean to be happy? In his book "The Art of Happiness," the Dalai Lama suggests that happiness has more to do with one's state of mind rather than external events. There is certainly much

1

wisdom in this idea; however, for teens who may be experiencing external events for the first time, they can take on a deeper significance. This is not to suggest that teenagers cannot understand the concept of how their state of mind can influence their happiness. It's pointing out that teens may not yet have the experience to engage with this idea and that the areas of the brain that are responsible for processing abstract ideas are still developing.

The Dalai Lama also suggests that all human beings have an innate desire to be happy and overcome suffering and that all humans have a fundamental right to pursue this state of being. I have found this to be true, that all the teenagers I have worked with have the desire to be happy and, for the most part, can get to that state.

The teenage years, with all of the physical and mental changes, changes in responsibility, expectations, relationships and social settings are an exciting and sometimes challenging time. The challenge and excitement of this time in life often brings with it emotional intensity. This intensity can also be characterized by rapid changes in mood, decision-making and response to various situations. With this intensity comes vast opportunity for connection, understanding and empowerment.

So what does a happy teen look like? Happiness is partly how you feel in general from day to day. It's also partly about how satisfied you are with things as they are and, to some degree, about what lies ahead. Happiness is about a state of mind, but also about how we respond to external events.

The teens I have worked with have talked to me about what it means for them to be happy and I'll share some of their thoughts below.

"When I'm happy, I just feel good. I'm not worried about anything. Even if I have things coming up, I don't think about them much."

"Being happy for me is feeling safe and cared about. It also means I am ready to laugh and have fun."

"Sometimes I'm happy on the inside, but my friends still ask me if something is wrong. I guess I don't always smile when I'm happy — at least not on the outside."

"I guess being happy is when I feel good inside and out. It's like when you're sick, it's not easy to be happy, even when I know I am going to get better."

Happiness is also influenced by our overall health. This doesn't mean you can't be sick and be happy. It does mean that being as healthy as possible affects your mood, emotions and ability to perform — not 30 years from now, but right now in this very second.

Health

What is health? Health is not simply the absence of disease or illness. It's sustaining a balance in mind, body and spirit. Our mind, body and spirit want to be whole and healthy and we can support or get in the way of that process.

Our bodies are truly amazing. If we stop to think about all the functions that happen within our bodies every day, every second, it's mind-boggling. Each second millions of cells die and are replaced, so in a way, we are new every second. This provides a unique opportunity to maintain and renew health.

Health is the coming together of many factors. It is difficult to be truly healthy if you focus only on having a healthy body or solely on building mental health. Both are important, but by themselves are limited. I am sure many of us have examples of people in our lives who look great and have healthy bodies but who are emotionally or mentally unhealthy. If we don't have them in our personal lives, we need look no further than professional athletes who can do amazing things with their bodies or entertainers who look wonderful and healthy, only to discover self-destructive practices as a result of neglecting other areas of their life.

The connection between the mind and body has been well-established for thousands of years. Indeed, many systems of health and medicine embrace and celebrate this idea. If there is any doubt about the connection between mind and body, close your eyes, take a few deep breaths and think about a situation or person that makes you angry for 30 seconds. Now notice the response in your body. Now, with our eyes still closed, take a few more deep breaths and think of a situation or person that makes you happy or that you find funny for 30 seconds. Notice the response in your body. It is likely that your body responded to both of those thoughts and responded in different ways.

In the first scenario, you may have felt anxious or like you wanted to get up and move. In the second scenario, you may have felt lighter in your limbs and chest. You may have felt excited and like you wanted to have that experience again. The fact that our minds and bodies are connected is a comforting thought and the healing power that this recognition has is empowering.

When it comes to health, there are different philosophies that people practice the world over. Below, I describe only a few in brief that I have suggested as part of an integrative approach.

In the Western world, we practice what is often called Western medicine, which, in general, will treat illnesses with pharmaceuticals or corrective surgery. Over the past few decades there has been more integration with other systems of medicine; namely, Traditional Chinese Medicine (TCM), incorporating such practices as acupuncture. Western medicine still tends to focus more on treating illnesses after the fact rather than prevention. There is also a tendency to view body, mind and spirit as separate rather than as an integrated whole.

Traditional Chinese Medicine (TCM) is a system of medicine developed in China that has been practiced for thousands of years. The general principles of TCM are that you are an integrated whole and every part of your body, mind and spirit are connected. Your body's systems do not function independently of each other. There is also a deep appreciation for our connection with the natural world and the role it plays in our health. TCM also recognizes your body's ability to heal itself and will often use treatments that will aid your body in healing itself.

In Traditional Chinese Medicine, there is a large focus on prevention; the idea that preventing illness in the first place is better than the best treatment. Traditional Chinese Medicine generally will use acupuncture, acupressure, Tuina massage, herbal therapy, dietary health and forms of energy work, such as Qi Gong, and exercise, such as Tai Chi, as the path to healing.

Another system of medicine that has been practiced for thousands of years is call Ayurvedic medicine or Ayurveda. Ayurveda originated in India approximately 5,000 years ago and its translation from Sanskrit means 'the science of life'. Ayurveda, like TCM, emphasizes the connection between mind, body sprit and our surroundings. The focus is on the balance of these areas in an effort to maintain vitality. One of the main foundations of Ayurveda is the belief that there are three basic energy patterns called doshas.

5

If you were to visit an Ayurvedic practitioner, he or she might prescribe breathing exercises to help promote relaxation and mindfulness, herbal medicine to restore balance, yoga and suggest ways of cleansing the body.

While going through every philosophy of medicine is well outside the scope of this book, I do want to mention Naturopathic medicine as another widely practiced system of wellness, focusing on treating the whole person and removing the causes of illness rather than just treating the symptoms.

What I have found is that using medicine and systems of wellness in an integrated fashion can be very powerful. Each system I have mentioned here contains aspects that it does very well. For instance, Western medicine has outstanding emergency and trauma care. Western medicine is also great for surgeries needed due to injury and has great physical therapy protocols. If I am ever in an accident, please take me to a trauma center, not an acupuncturist or a naturopath. However, after I have been stabilized, I might employ a mixture of acupuncture, breathing, diet and physical therapy, as well as some herbal therapies to reduce inflammation and heal.

It has also been my finding that Western medicine is a bit too quick to prescribe medications to treat the symptoms of illness, especially when it comes to ADD, ADHD, anxiety, depression and simple teenage emotion. Often these medications have harmful side effects such as heart palpitations, headaches, drowsiness, loss of appetite, irritability, confusion and loss of body control. With that being said, there are times where medication is warranted and helpful.

Now, to be clear, I am not recommending that anyone refuse to take medications prescribed by their healthcare professional. What I am saying is to research, ask questions and talk to your medical professional about trying methods other than medication, such as dietary modifications, breathing techniques, yoga, etc., initially.

So what does it mean to be a happy/healthy teen? As we know, the teen years are a time of rapid change and growth. Just think of the changes between ages 13 and 18. I always say knowledge, especially self-knowledge, is empowering. Knowing that the teen years are a time of rapid change and that being happy and healthy are tied together, teens can take charge of this process and adults can support teens as they take charge; that's the first step.

In the coming chapters, we will go through different areas of health and happiness while exploring the real-life experiences of the teenagers I have worked with, all the time looking at ways of integrating different areas of health and happiness.

You are not expected to be and need not be an expert in the various systems of medicine and wellness, but are invited to explore with an open heart and mind ways to maintain health and happiness. Ultimately, you will make the choice on what to use, what to disregard and what to modify to fit your needs. In the words of Bruce Lee, "Adapt what is useful, reject what is useless and add what is specifically your own."

Chapter Two

Challenges To Teen Health & Happiness

Young people are in the midst of an unprecedented health crisis. For the first time, young people have ailments that used to be limited to adults. From physical health issues, such as obesity and diabetes, to mental health issues, such as ADD and depression, what today's young people are facing can conservatively be considered a crisis.

According to the Centers for Disease Control (2013), childhood obesity has doubled in young children and tripled in adolescents in the past 30 years. Type 2 diabetes, a disease normally seen in adults over 40, is on the rise in children and adolescents (Centers for Disease Control, 2013). The number of cases of nonalcoholic fatter liver disease in young people over the age of 10 is on the rise (Vajro et al., 2012).

These are not the only health issues today's young people are faced with, as mental health disorders such as anxiety, depression, bipolar and mood disorders are prevalent in adolescents and young adults. The World Health Organization (2012) estimates that 20 percent of adolescents worldwide experience a mental health problem every year.

Add in the approximately 3.5 million young people that are taking medications for Attention Deficit Disorder (ADD) and Attention Deficit Hyperactivity Disorder (ADHD) and the fact that some estimates suggest that half of young people, ages 10 to 21, in the United States have some form of learning disability, it's no wonder that many young people today feel confused, out of touch with themselves and powerless to do anything to change their situation.

Young people are often confused by the mixed messages they receive about health from the media, family, friends and society at large. On one hand, they are shown unrealistic images of lean-muscled female and male bodies that are airbrushed and/or touched up to hide imperfections as the ultimate in health. These images are confusing, unrealistic and represent a limited view of health. While the people in these images may indeed be healthy, we have no real way of knowing if they really are.

On the other hand, young people are told to be healthy and that being healthy is important, yet they are surrounded by a sea of junk, imitations and distorted views of life that are available 24 hours a day. Teens are bombarded with advertising images specifically developed for their age group with their developmental needs, wants and desires factored in. The morality of this is a topic for a later time; however, I will say that using the knowledge of how a still-developing mind processes information can be used for higher or better purposes.

Through technology — social media and mobile apps alone — teens can be exposed to hundreds of ads per day. If we take other daily activities into account, this number soars into the thousands. Teens are targeted simply because they are major consumers of certain products and generally have not yet developed brand loyalty. However, if you have some sort of emotional connection to a product as a child, you are more likely to stay with that product as an adult; in other words, you become a lifelong user of that product.

As we can imagine, the ads teens are most likely to see are not designed to give them healthy choices. They are designed to convince them to buy and consume a product, hopefully for life. It matters little whether they spend their own or someone else's money (e.g., parent, guardian) or what the cost to their overall health and happiness is.

A recent conversation I had with a group of teens on this subject went something like this, "We know that media is filled with advertisements made by people who are paid to figure out ways to sell us stuff. Even though I know it, sometimes I still feel like I might be missing something or that someone may have something that I should have. Whoever these people are, they are good at making us think we need their stuff or that we should do what they tell us we should do."

Another unhealthy side of media — in particular, social media — is that it has become a dumping ground for everyone's opinions and beliefs and a forum to spread hate, intolerance and falsehoods. Many groups have adopted social media as their platform to spread their own brand of facts, whether they are well researched or not. It can be overwhelming and confusing to sift through all the rhetoric and propaganda. It's not often people's minds are changed by a discussion on social media.

Ray, a teenager I chatted with some months back, put it this way, "It's like I don't know who to believe or trust on social media. Everyone says they are right and that the other people are lying. It's like some people go on there just to say crazy things or maybe just to argue. I hear my parents say that teenagers don't care about the world. I think it's just hard to because we see all this stuff on social media and we don't know what to do."

Today's teens are certainly aware and savvy when it comes to peer pressure. Even with the knowledge of how powerful peer pressure can be and the constant encouragement to be yourself, go against the grain and not follow the crowd, the need we all have to fit in, to be accepted or to have a social network can be a strong driving force. This drive is especially strong in the teen years when one's sense of belonging or being part of a group seems as necessary to survival as food and water.

I don't want to paint an absolute negative picture of peer pressure because it can be and is positive when it's about being encouraged to take care of yourself. Peer pressure can range from friends pestering you to go out and eat fast food, to go to a movie instead of studying, to stay up late and not get enough sleep, to the pressure to take drugs, drink alcohol and drive, to have sex when you're not ready and/or to commit a crime or violence. Peer pressure makes it easier to develop unhealthy patterns of behavior.

Reading this you may think, what's the big deal about eating fast food or staying up late? In the short term, maybe not that much, but eating fast food and staying up late affects you right now. The need to be socially accepted is certainly a trait that all humans share. We all like to take part in behaviors or rituals that make us feel connected or a part of something. Teens have a strong desire to be with their peer group and feel a part of that group. It really does look like all teens want to do is be with their friends and have little time for all else. The pressure that comes with this need is powerful.

"Some days all I want to do is see and talk to my friends. We do get to text each other a lot or Zoom or Skype, so it's usually not that bad if I don't get to see them."

"Yeah, I do think my friends push me to do things that I don't always want to do or really never thought about doing. It even happens with kids who aren't really my friends. I usually don't feel good about it after, but I know that I don't always just follow what everyone else is doing either."

While being part of a group is great, let's be mindful of the challenges peer pressure can present in terms of health and happiness.

Technology

While a good number of teens feel they are technologically literate and are able to leverage it in a variety of ways, many still express feeling disconnected from each other and the world. So as technology has the capacity to connect us, there seems to be something missing. Technology can also become a distraction and it makes it easy to disengage from more personal interactions.

Technology becomes a challenge to teen health and happiness when it gets in the way of personal interactions, is used as a way to avoid connecting or becomes the sole activity. The phrase 'sitting is the new smoking' should give teens pause about the detrimental effects prolonged sitting has on our health, and technology certainly has made it easier to sit for long periods of time.

When you don't have to get up to entertain yourself and when, literally, the world is at your fingertips, you don't have to move to get an experience. Yes, I am aware that there are games and interactive apps and videos that require movement. These are great if they are incorporated into a daily routine.

We know that technology can be extremely useful, but it presents a unique challenge in that, in a very real way if one doesn't use some form of technology in today's world, it's an impediment to communication and, to some degree, learning. On the other hand, it tends to force us to sit and be inactive and remain indoors and to rely on it for communication and interaction.

How many times have we sent a text or an e-mail when a phone call or an in-person chat would have been best? E-mail and texting can be great ways to stay in touch with our friends and loved ones; however, there is a lot that can get misinterpreted in text or e-mail. I believe this is where the feeling of disconnection starts. What is said in a text or an e-mail can take on a bigger meaning than what it was intended to. All too often it results in hurt feelings, misunderstandings and strained relationships. Technology also brings with it the challenges that social media presents, as discussed above.

Technology will likely increase in the years to come in terms of access and capability. For teens — and really all of us — it will continue to be a useful tool as well as a challenge to our health and happiness if we let it be.

Too Much Structure

"I know my friends feel the same way. We have too much to do and not enough time to do it." Of course, we can hear this same lament from adults, but to hear it from teens who, in my opinion, need much more unstructured time, is concerning. During this important developmental stage, time for reflection is critical.

I have heard many arguments for the justification of this need to have every minute scheduled. None, in my experience, hold water. Even in the short term overscheduling can present challenges to teen health and happiness. One challenge is the time to get enough sleep and rest. Sleep deprivation can cause serious health issues as well as immediate impact to focus, attention span, ability to reason, along with irritability and mood swings. It's difficult to feel happy when you are sleep deprived.

Having too much structure also leads to a reduced ability to be comfortable with uncertainty or lack of structure. I can't tell you how often I hear adults express their concern that so many teens are so used to having every minute planned and structured that they have a hard time functioning without it.

The problem is not with structure; the problem is with too much structure. When everything is scheduled, a lot of energy is spent running from one activity to another with little time to stop and enjoy each activity. The experience is a bit more superficial when you run from one activity to another without any time to stop, think and reflect.

The argument I hear most often is that, 'It's best for teens to be busy, otherwise they will get into trouble.' First, the negative view of teens in this statement is concerning. Second, being busy isn't necessarily bad; boredom can be worse. Being too busy and having too much structure can lead to anxiety, stress and depression. Too much structure can also kill creativity.

As I chatted with a group of teens about how much structure they had in their lives, I asked them to map out what a typical week looks like for them. I was stunned at the results. While everyone's schedule was a little different in terms of what they were doing, they differed little in their actual daily schedules.

This is what a typical weekday schedule looked like:

5:45 am - Wake up

6:30 am - 5:30 pm - Getting to school, school, after-school activities (including sports and clubs)

5:30 pm - 7:30 pm - Music, marital arts, gymnastics lessons, town team sports

7:30 - 8:30 - Shower, eat dinner

8:30 - ??? - Homework, get ready for the next day

The group reported that their weekend schedule was, in general, tightly scheduled. Between games, practices, meetings and family obligations, the overall feeling was that there was little downtime. This schedule is difficult to sustain.

It is wonderful that teens have many choices of what they can engage in, and I, personally, recommend taking advantage of having the time to explore different interest areas. We also need to seriously consider what the right amount of structure is.

Access To Healthy Choices

As teenagers move more towards independence, they make more and more decisions for themselves. The choices that they make, in part, have to do with access. If all you have access to are choices that are unhealthy, then it's a next-to-impossible task to make healthy choices.

Of course, more than just access determines the choices teens make. What I have found is that if the choices are there, teens will at least consider them. Teens and adults can work together to make sure that teens have access to plenty of healthy choices. When teens do not have access to affordable options for entertainment and leisure activities or a safe place where they can gather, it makes it difficult to have social interactions outside of structured time.

It's important for teens to have access to choices for their health care that take their whole being into account. In Chapter One, I mentioned some different philosophies and approaches to healthcare and prevention. When teens either do not know about or are not given access to a variety of ways to balance their health and happiness, this can have a negative effect.

Perhaps the most important is having access to whole, healthy foods. The lack of access to whole, healthy foods may be one of the biggest contributors to the challenges teens face when it comes to their health and happiness. In the next chapter, I go into much more detail about nutrition, whole foods and the impact they have on teen health and happiness.

It is true that teens do have many challenges to overcome when it comes to being healthy and happy and some of the challenges are just in day-to-day living. And there is good news! Throughout the rest of this book, I share what I have found works for teens in overcoming these challenges — and not just overcoming, but being empowered to take charge of their health and their lives.

Chapter Three

Nutrition

We truly are what we eat. While there are experts who will dispute this claim, I have found that what you eat and drink can and often does have an immediate impact on how you feel, your mood and how you perform. An example of this is the feeling of being hungry, irritable, tired or having a hard time concentrating within hours or minutes of consuming high amounts of sugar or carbohydrates.

I am not a nutritionist, nor do I claim to be, yet I have witnessed the positive effects making even small adjustments to eating can have and has had for the teens I have worked with. I have had the experience of watching the opposite hold true as well.

Does this mean you can never have a chip, a cookie, a candy bar, fast food, ice cream, pizza or a soda? No, it doesn't. And the additional good news is that there are healthy or healthier versions of these treats readily available. At the end of the chapter, I provide healthy suggestions along with a few teen-approved recipes that are simple, nutritious, delicious and fun to prepare.

There are literally hundreds of dietary theories out there all claiming to have the science to back them up. We are also surrounded by food — or food-like substances — and in many parts of the world they are available 24-7. As we found out in Chapter Two, there is a lot of money and effort spent on marketing these food-like substances to teens. Indeed, it is now possible to never leave your home and have food or food-like substances delivered to you whenever you want them.

So what do we do? Who do we listen to? Should I eat Paleo or raw vegan? While this book is not about promoting any one dietary theory or way of eating, what follows below are a few common threads that I have found throughout the most well-researched theories and what I have found to work well for teens.

Enjoy Your Food

One of the best things we can do is enjoy our food, even if the food we are eating isn't the best choice for us. If you decide to indulge, then do it with gusto. I am not advocating overeating or frequent indulgence. What I am saying is that we should enjoy our food. And if you decide to eat those potato chips, then enjoy them guilt-free. The stress of worrying can sometimes be more damaging than the actual indulgence itself.

Balance Is Key

Balancing your meals with good fats, lean proteins, vegetables and good carbohydrates is important. Another part of the idea of balance is to balance out your indulgences with good choices. For instance, if you ate junk food all day on Saturday, perhaps on Sunday you would eat only fruits, vegetables, good fats and lean proteins. You would also opt for lighter meals. You can even do this from meal to meal. If you indulged at breakfast, simply make lunch and dinner healthier, lighter meals.

Whole foods are foods that are as close to their natural state as possible with minimal processing. An example of this would be eating an apple rather than a slice of apple pie or even applesauce, which are often loaded with sugar and artificial ingredients.

Why choose whole foods? Whole foods, such as blueberries, wild-caught salmon, nuts and seeds (such as walnuts, almonds and sunflower seeds), avocados, whole grains (oatmeal, millet and quinoa), dark chocolate (cacao), green vegetables (kale, broccoli, celery) and pomegranates help specifically with memory and concentration, not to mention overall brain health.

Additionally, whole foods are likely to contain a combination of good fats, phytochemicals like antioxidants, fiber and a high degree of nutrients. Nutrients taken in by eating whole foods are more easily utilized by the body. Eating whole foods ensures the most efficient usage of nutrients that fuel brain activity, such as concentration, focus, memory and problem solving and also have a positive effect on emotions and stress. Of course, nutrients are used to fuel more than just the activity of our brains, they are used to sustain the functions of our body.

Choose Foods High In Nutrients

Nutrients range from the macros, such as carbohydrates, fats and proteins, to micros, such as vitamins and minerals. In general, macronutrients are what are bodies require in higher amounts and micronutrients are what we require in smaller amounts. However, while we may require smaller amounts of micronutrients, a real deficiency in micronutrients, such as iron, iodine and zinc, can have serious health consequences, as they allow our bodies to produce enzymes, hormones and other substances that are vital to healthy functioning (Micronutrient Facts, 2015).

Choosing foods that are highest in nutrients, sometimes referred to as nutrient density, ensures that we are providing our body with what it needs in a way that's easy for it to use. When we complicate this process by, say, eating foods that are highly processed or that contain additives, it causes our bodies to have to work harder to discard what it cannot use or work harder to make the little use that it can of these nutrient-deficient foods.

Some great nutrient-dense foods are:

- Wild-caught salmon
- Kale
- Raw garlic
- Sprouts
- Liver from grass-fed, pasture-raised beef

Good Fats

We need to eat fat for our bodies to function well. Among many of its benefits are that it's a good source of energy, it's needed for cell-wall building and is essential in immune system functioning. There is much research on the connection between high-quality fats — especially Omega 3s — and the function of nerve cells, synapses (the spaces in between nerve cells that carry chemical signals) and the health of our myelin sheath, which acts as a protective covering to our nerve cells.

What Are Good Fats?

Monounsaturated fats are plant-based fats and, in general, are considered to be a healthy source of fat. Monounsaturated fats are found in foods like avocados, black and green olives, nuts like almonds and macadamia nuts, nut butters and oils like olive oil.

Polyunsaturated fats are Omega 3 and Omega 6 fatty acids, which are also called essential fatty acids and are types of polyunsaturated fats that we cannot make in our bodies. We need to get them from the food we eat. These fats are needed for healthy brain and nerve function, for healthy skin and mucous membranes, to reduce bad cholesterol (LDL) and increase good cholesterol (HDL), as well as having many other health benefits. Good sources of Omega 3s are fatty fish like wild-caught salmon and mackerel, flaxseeds and walnuts. Good sources of Omega 6s are nuts and seeds. You need more Omega 3s than Omega 6s, so avoid using oils that are high in Omega 6s.

Saturated fats are fats that are found in animal products as well as in coconut and palm oils. Saturated fat has recently had a bit of a resurgence, as the health benefits of saturated fats are being recognized. While saturated fats are necessary for strong bones, healthy immune system and brain functioning, you don't have to get them from animal products and they should make up the smallest amount of the fats that you take in.

Bad Fats

Trans fats are fats that are taken from liquid form and turned into solid form. They are turned into solids by adding in hydrogen atoms. This expands their shelf life. You should avoid these as much as possible because they contain little to no nutritional value and can cause weight gain, raise bad cholesterol and lower good cholesterol, raise your risk of diabetes, affect brain function and cause inflammation.

Many processed foods contain added trans fats, especially any food that contains partially-hydrogenated oils. Trans fats are also in foods that are fried in partially-hydrogenated oils like French fries and doughnuts, in margarines and in shortenings and in baked goods like crackers, cookies and pies.

Fermented Foods

In short, fermented foods are foods that are left to sit to increase the beneficial bacteria and helpful enzymes that are contained in these foods. Fermented foods have incredible health benefits and have become synonymous with the term 'good bacteria' or 'probiotics'.

The probiotics in fermented foods are pretty much essential for good gut or intestinal health. It's been said that our immune-system health starts with our gut and, in particular, the amount of good bacteria in our gut. Our gut health is linked to our overall health and has been linked to behavior, weight gain/loss and good digestion, as it helps us absorb the nutrients from the food we eat.

Fiber

Fiber, sometimes called roughage, is basically the part of plants that we are not able to fully digest. It helps move food through our digestive system. Some important health benefits of fiber are that it promotes normal bowel movements, bowel health, lowers cholesterol levels and helps us to maintain a healthy weight. Fiber is found in grains, legumes, seeds, fruit and vegetables.

Fruits & Vegetables

It turns out that your grandmother was right; eat vegetables and fruits as much as you can. Eating fruits and vegetables is probably the best way to get a lot of good nutrients into your body. Some fruits are high in sugar, so it's best to eat those in moderation.

I could probably fill a whole book with the benefits of fruits and vegetables, as many lower blood pressure, reduce the risk of heart disease, prevent certain types of cancers, promote mental clarity and maintain a healthy weight. Eat a variety of fruits and vegetables as much as you can and mix the colors. Some vegetables and fruits that have high nutrient density are kale, watercress, collard greens, broccoli, lemons, strawberries, blueberries and blackberries.

Bio-Individuality

Every person has a unique ecosystem inside of them. While there are certainly some healthy practices — things that are common to all of us —

each of us is different and what works for one person may not work for another. I advise getting to know your unique makeup and what works for you and seeking out medical practitioners that will get to know your bio-individuality and continue to learn about what works uniquely for you.

Limit Processed Foods/Foods With Many Additives And Ingredients

Processed foods are basically any foods that are changed in some way before we eat them. It can be a simple change like drying or freezing to complex changes where the food hardly resembles its original form.

Often foods that are highly processed are loaded with additives and artificial ingredients. There are many reasons for this; mostly it's about making these products last a long time and making them taste good enough for you to want to eat and keep eating them. The food additive industry is a billions-of-dollars-a-year industry.

Processed foods are usually pretty easy to distinguish from whole foods. For example, blueberry breakfast pastries, which are often loaded with processed sugar and many artificial chemicals and additives, would not be considered a whole food, as opposed to real blueberries, which are a whole food.

So what's the problem with processed foods? So what if they have more additives and are processed. Let's take the example above. Eating this 'food' may actually dull memory and concentration in the short run and in the long run may lead to brain deficiencies as well as other negative health effects. In short, processed foods and foods with many additives can have adverse effects on teen health and happiness.

Come on, isn't eating junk food a right of passage for teenagers? Isn't this the time when they should be doing it? Do we really want to take away this freedom from them?

Yes, one of the many wonderful things about being a teenager is that you can consume foods that would cause most adults serious weight gain or other issues; however, this does not mean teenagers are immune to the negative effects of junk food. Just look at the rates of obesity, diabetes (Centers for Disease Control, 2013) and other diseases that were normally relegated to adults (Vajro et al., 2012).

I want to be clear that there is food and there is junk. Junk food really is a misnomer. We are certainly surrounded by food-like substances, but that doesn't make them food. Junk food is basically a food-like substance that has minute to no nutritional value and adds a lot of calories to one's diet. These are known as empty calories and are much of the cause of weight gain and other challenges to teen health and happiness.

It is generally easy to spot junk food. It is the most processed, packaged food with long lists of ingredients and additives that are not created for the purposes of nutrition and generally do not take any preparation on one's part to consume like chips, cookies, crackers, candy and prepackaged meals.

The good news is that there are healthy or healthier alternatives available, which we will discuss at the end of this chapter.

Sugar

There is natural sugar (fructose, glucose, lactose, maltose, sucrose) found in fruits and plants, and refined sugar, which puts unusable forms of raw sugar through processing so that it is usable. What is left after the processing is refined sugar without any nutrients or vitamins and is just basically empty calories. While there are some who disagree, conventional wisdom from most experts is that refined sugar should make up a minuscule amount of your daily calories and even should be avoided entirely.

Some of the negative effects of sugar include heart damage, weight gain, production of cancer cells, foggy thinking, overloading of the liver, can cause insulin resistance, is highly addictive, interferes with immune function, promotes tooth decay, gum disease, accelerates aging, affects behavior, increases stress, causes headaches, mood swings and can reduce brain capacity. Refined sugar can also strip the body of vitamins and minerals.

Teenagers are more susceptible to the effects of sugar than adults. Sugar can change blood flow to the still-developing parts of the teenage brain and has been shown to increase the stress response in teens, which can exacerbate anxiety and depression.

Part of the challenge is that refined sugar shows up under many different names, such as evaporated cane juice and basically anything that ends with an 'ose' or has the word 'syrup' in it. Also challenging is that refined sugar shows up in products that might surprise you. This, along with the advertising directed at teens to get them to consume food and drink that are high in sugar, and it's easy for teens to fall into the sugar trap.

Again, there is good news that there are sweeteners that we can use that are healthier choices. I will go into more detail at the end of the chapter, but a couple that are easy to get and use are stevia and xylitol. A note of caution: Just because these may be healthier options doesn't mean it's a good idea to overdo it.

Condiments/Sauces

Many of us love to have a condiment or sauce to go along with our food or we like to cook with particular sauces. Sauces and condiments are the same as food in that there are options that are healthy or healthier and ones that have negative impacts on our health. Condiments and sauces are where a lot of hidden sugar shows up. Who would think that ketchup and barbecue sauce contain sugar? In fact, sometimes they are made up of mostly sugar.

Like food, choosing condiments and sauces that have the most nutritional value and the least amount of additives and refined sugar whenever possible is a good rule of thumb.

Sugary Drinks/Energy Drinks

These are often loaded with so much sugar that really they are sugar with some other added ingredients. In these drinks, other ingredients range from dyes or colorings to aspartame in soft drinks to caffeine and taurine in energy drinks.

Twelve ounces of many sodas contain 39 grams of refined sugar. The popular 20-ounce size contains 65 grams of refined sugar. The same goes for many of the fruit juices we come across, as they are often made by the same companies that bring us the sugary sodas and energy drinks. Many of these fruit juices have the same amount of or even more sugar per ounce than soda.

I don't think I am overstating it when I say that these types of drinks are probably one of the biggest culprits that negatively impact teen health and happiness and they are one of the easiest things to change.

I have seen dramatic shifts in teen mental and physical health just by avoiding or cutting down on these drinks. If you are a teen struggling with weight and find that you drink a lot of these types of drinks, try cutting back or avoiding them altogether and see what that does for you.

Organic Food

Organic food or food grown organically is food that is grown without the use of chemical pesticides, synthetic fertilizers, sewage sludge or GMO's. Organic animal products come from animals, in general, that are not given antibiotics or growth hormones and are fed organic feed and/or are pasture raised.

There is still debate and controversy over whether organic food is better for you. The organic and conventional sides claim the other has conducted shoddy or flawed research or has ulterior motives in taking a stance one way or the other. Despite these sideswipes and the continual back and forth, my opinion is that organic food is worth the expense and the effort. I have witnessed noticeable differences when teens I have worked with switched to eating more organic foods.

There is no question that organic food is quite often more expensive than food that is conventionally grown. The good news is that organic food is becoming more affordable and available. Many locations have farmer's markets and/or CSAs (Community Supported Agriculture) and these are great

28

ways to get organic, local-grown food that is in season; another aspect that I highly recommend.

We also have the option of buying what The Environmental Working Group calls the 'Clean 15', which are foods that, while conventionally grown, are grown with the least amount of pesticides. This does not account for whether synthetic fertilizers are used.

Whether or not organic food is an option, it is still best to eat whole foods, organic or not.

Water

The human brain is made up largely of water. Drinking plenty of clean, plain water helps keep the brain well hydrated and functioning at an optimal level. Many studies have shown that drinking water aids in brain functioning and that lack of brain hydration leads to most temporary difficulties in concentration and focus.

There is some debate over how much water is enough, whether we need to get all of our water from drinking it or could we get it from a combination of drinking and eating foods with a high water content. While bodies differ in this requirement, a safe estimate is to drink six to eight glasses of water per day. This also depends on the outside temperature and your activity level.

Since, as we know, the teenage brain is still developing and doing so at a rapid rate, drinking water and keeping the brain hydrated becomes even more important. Water is also essential for physical performance, gives us more energy, keeps our bowels healthy, is good for our skin, helps to oxygenate our blood and keeps muscles and joints elastic.

It is a good idea to carry a water bottle with you that you can drink from throughout the day. A glass water bottle with a protective cover is a great option, since it easy to clean and there are no worries about toxins leaching into the water. Stainless steel water bottles are also a great choice. Clean, filtered water is generally the best choice. There is really no need to buy bottled water unless for some reason you do not have access to clean water or your water is somehow contaminated.

Anything added to the water is just another substance the body has to break down. If there is an intense aversion to drinking plain water, try adding a tiny amount of stevia to sweeten it a bit or a small amount of low-sugar, 100% organic not-from-concentrate fruit juice with no additives, such as apple or cranberry. You can decrease this amount weekly until finally you're drinking just plain water.

There are many other benefits to drinking water and we have barely scratched the surface here. A final thing I will say about the importance of water to our bodies is that we can survive roughly between 30 to 40 days without food and only three to four days without water.

What Is Put On The Body

Our skin is the largest organ in our body. Much of what we put on our skin can be absorbed into our bloodstream. While I am keeping this part short, it is no less important in terms of teen health and happiness.

If we are paying close attention and care to what is taken *into* the body through eating and drinking, the same attention must be given to what is put *on* the body. In the same way that what is put in the body can have a positive or negative impact on teen health and happiness, the same goes for what is put on the body.

So what we put on our body is just as important as what we put in it and the same reasoning we use to decide what we put in it can be applied to what we put on it. In short, if you can't put it in your mouth, it shouldn't go on your skin. It takes only 26 seconds for anything that is put on your body to be absorbed through your skin and end up in your bloodstream. Instead of using toxic products on your body, there are many effective, nontoxic alternatives to choose from.

So What Do We Do Now?

All this is great, Pete, but what do I do now? This is what I have often heard from teens and parents. My answer has always been and remains that, yes, there seems to be a lot to do, but it doesn't have to be difficult or stressful. In fact, it should be enjoyable.

There is certainly a lot of information here and it can seem to be a bit daunting, so the best place for us to start is by going through some questions together.

These questions are not about a right or wrong answer. Don't worry about what you think the answers are supposed to be; just answer as honestly as you can. It's about bringing awareness to what is happening and having time for reflection. You may find that just answering these questions provides new insight or a new perspective.

Whether you're a teen or adult reading this book, the questions are here to get you to think about what you are taking into your body. If you're an adult that isn't a parent to teens but works with teens, answer the questions based on what you have observed from working with teens.

So grab a piece of paper and a pen, get comfortable, sit back, relax and have fun answering the following questions:

- *Question 1:* What is/are the teen/s in your life's current nutrition like? It may be helpful to map out a typical day of meals. I recommend choosing two days; one weekday and one weekend day.

- *Question 2:* Based on your answer to Question 1, what are some areas of nutrition that are going particularly well? What are some areas that can improve?

- *Question 3:* Which foods make up the biggest portion of the teen/s in your life's diet? For example, do they eat a lot of chicken, lots of cauliflower, lots of cookies, crackers, processed foods, etc.?

- *Question 4:* Based on your answers to the last three questions, do the areas that are going well make up the biggest portion of their diet?

- *Question 5:* What is the biggest challenge to the teen/s in your life eating whole, nutrient-dense, organic, minimally-processed foods with minimal ingredients?

I suggest revisiting these questions from time to time to note any changes and to see your progress. I offer the following recommendations based on my work with teens in the field that will help with the answers to the above questions. I also provide some examples of how these recommendations have been and are being used.

Keep It Simple

Michael Pollan has three simple "Food Rules" that I think keep things simple when it comes to thinking about the food choices we make. I recommend reading or watching anything that was created by Michael Pollan.

Here are a few "Food Rules" from his work that I have found to work really well:

- ✓ Eat whole foods
- ✓ Mostly plants
- ✓ Not too much

Here are a few more "Food Rules" from his work that I have found to work really well:

- ✓ Eat things with less than five ingredients
- ✓ Only eat things that will eventually rot
- ✓ Don't buy food where you buy your gas

Try not to overthink every choice related to what you eat. If you find yourself surrounded by poor choices, you can still make the best choice possible. One possibility is to skip eating until you can get to a place where you have better choices. Certainly, I am not recommending skipping meals on a regular basis, but once in a while will not hurt you and may be your best option.

"It's hard for me to keep this all straight in my head. I think I know what to do, but then I am not always sure." This is what Ray, a junior in high school, told me when we talked about nutrition. We started out with the "Food Rules" from Michael Pollan and worked with each one and individualized them in a way that worked for him. The biggest challenge for Ray was finding the right mixture of plant-based foods that he enjoyed and also could find easily.

We started with building on the things that he liked, such as tomatoes, cucumbers and lettuce, and then introduced in other plant-based foods that were easy to get, such as carrots, spinach and celery. Once we started mixing these foods together, we branched out to other foods. We kept it simple and found what worked. I recommend you do the same.

"Let Food Be Thy Medicine And Let Medicine Be Thy Food"

You may have come across this quote from Hippocrates somewhere along the way. While I think some take this too literally, what we eat can help us feel better and aid in healing. I want to be clear, I am not suggesting that medication or other forms of healing should not be used, but rather that nutrition can be a big factor in how we feel, function and heal.

Think about it in this way: If you aren't feeling well and consume processed foods with a long list of ingredients and additives, your body now has to work harder to break these down and that takes away energy it could be using for healing your body and another way to think about it is taking in foods that will give your body the most nourishment when you are not feeling your best.

Amanda was about a year into her teenage years when she and her parents came to me. Amanda was experiencing major anxiety and stated that she was starting to have panic attacks. She had been to see the family physician, who prescribed her medication. In her words, "As soon as I started taking it, I felt out of it and I have no energy." Her parents reported that she seemed depressed and even with the medication the anxiety was still there.

While we worked on more than just nutrition alone, her nutrition is one of the first places we started. What we found was that Amanda and her family were eating a lot of highly processed takeout food. Also, Amanda seemed to have a significant love of anything sweet, along with energy drinks that she consumed daily.

Often when anxiety is the issue, there is a deficiency in magnesium. Looking at what Amanda was consuming on daily basis, it was clear that she was not getting enough magnesium, along with consuming artificial dyes, additives and caffeine in the form of energy drinks. These all were contributing to her anxiety, panic attacks and depression. When we slowly introduced more foods like dark leafy greens, nuts, seeds, fish, beans, whole grains and avocados into her diet that contain magnesium, her symptoms started to lessen. We also used some supplements and oils to help bring up her magnesium levels and work with some other deficiencies.

Eventually, Amanda's physician took her off the medication she had originally been on. "I know that paying attention to what I eat has helped me. I don't freak out about it, but I do pay attention."

Yes, I do recommend supplements, herbs and essential oils. Of course, before starting to use any of these you would want to consult with your healthcare professional. I recommend treating these in the same way that you treat food. Only use high-quality, whole-food supplements, herbs and essential oils that do not contain artificial flavors, synthetics, colors, dyes or sugars.

As in the case of Amanda above, we used a magnesium and vitamin D supplement, along with magnesium oil and lavender essential oil. The magnesium oil could be applied directly to the skin in small amounts and the lavender essential oil was used aromatically in a diffuser.

"I'll rip your freaking head off! Get away from me!" is what Jake would say to many of his teachers. He also could and did get violent to the point where he would throw things, knock or turn things over or get physical with someone. So when I had my first conversation with Jake over the phone, I could tell just from that conversation that he was in an agitated, aggressive state.

When we finally met, I could see he was agitated to the point where it was hard for him to sit still and he always seemed on the verge of going into a rage. Jake said a few times during this meeting that he felt like he wanted to rip his skin off. He also told me that he didn't sleep much, that he really didn't know why he would get angry and have the outbursts described above and that he was upset at himself for gaining so much weight.

Two things that I cued in on was Jake's reference to gaining a lot of weight and Jake's mother telling me that some blood work they had recently had done showed that Jake's vitamins B and D levels were very low. One of the first things we did was to get Jake on high-quality, whole-food B and D vitamin supplements. Within a few days, Jake's behavior went from a ten to about a six, which was a marked improvement. This allowed Jake to feel more grounded and took away the feeling of wanting to rip out of his skin.

This allowed conversations to take place around food and other issues in which we found that Jake had sensitivities to certain foods. When those foods were minimized or avoided, Jake's behavior continued to improve. Taking supplements and avoiding certain foods were not the only things that we worked on together; however, I believe that using these first opened the door to doing the continued work that we did. It wouldn't have happened without them.

Pay Attention To Digestion

You can eat whole, nutritious, unprocessed, organic foods, but if you cannot digest or absorb them, you will not be receiving much of the benefits. Proper digestion is a key to health and happiness. It may be uncomfortable to talk about, but digestion helps you break down your food into the nutrients your body needs and also helps to eliminate waste properly. I can't tell you how many teens I have worked with that have had a digestive issue or poor digestion. It's not something that, as a teen, you would think about often unless there is a real problem; however, even minor issues build over time and can affect health and happiness.

Think about being constipated frequently or not being able to eliminate regularly and how that makes you feel. How often one should eliminate or poop varies on the person. In general, the normal range is anywhere from three times a day to three times a week. I've found that eliminating at least once a day has a positive impact on health and happiness.

When there are digestive issues, a change in diet that includes more fruits and vegetables and introducing digestive enzymes, along with fermented foods, to one's diet can help to improve digestion. I have had teens say that once their digestion improves, they feel lighter and less toxic.

Keep A Food Journal

One of the easiest ways to get a handle on your nutrition is to keep a food journal. You can make this as complex or as simple as you like. It can be just a record of your meals, simply writing what you ate and drank and what the ingredients were. You can also get more complex and note how you felt right after eating the meal and again a few hours later. You can also write about changes in your mood, hunger level and overall general feelings. The idea is to notice any patterns and make adjustments based on the patterns. Again, this is not about beating yourself up if you find that you need to make some improvements, it's about getting to know yourself and how you may react to certain foods.

By keeping a food journal, you may notice that you have a sensitivity to certain foods or drinks. In fact, some teens I have worked with only wrote in their food journal when they noticed a change after eating certain foods. This helped us hone in on some of the problem areas.

"I remember when you first talked to me about doing this, I really didn't see the point. I thought journals were for writing down feelings or talking about my day. Now I think the food journal really helped. It helped me think about the food I was eating and how it could change how I felt."

I remember working with Luis, who had started to feel depressed and, as he called it, 'too moody'. Through using the food journal, we noticed that part of the reason for his depression is that he felt he had no control over what he was eating and that he was overwhelmed by trying to figure out how and what to eat.

Read Labels

Learning to read labels can be empowering. I, personally, believe that everyone has a right to know what's in their food and where it comes from. When it comes to reading labels, look for foods that have five ingredients or less. If what you pick up has a long list of ingredients and has things like artificial coloring, dyes and a long list of chemical additives or words you can't pronounce, it is not the best choice.

The first listed ingredient is generally what it contains the most of, so if the first ingredient listed is sugar, then you will be consuming mostly sugar or a large amount of it. If the first ingredient says grapes, then that's what it is mostly made up of. Be careful though, because even foods that list something like grapes first can still have a long list of ingredients that include artificial colors, flavors and other chemical additives. A good rule of thumb is that if you can't recognize the ingredients or you're not quite sure what they are, then don't eat it, at least until you can find out what those ingredients are.

You also may come across something called fractionated oils or partially-hydrogenated oils. It is best to completely avoid these or minimize their intake as much as possible. You will find these in most snack foods and many other processed foods. They are chemically unstable in the body and create free radicals, which are cancer-causing agents. There are healthier choices out there.

Read labels to know what you're eating.

Get Involved With/Prepare Your Own Food

This may be the most powerful way to take control of what you eat. You don't have to be dependent on 'fast food' or someone else to make your meals. It also gives you more of a connection with where your food comes from and what goes into preparing it. Not everyone aspires to be a professional chef or wants to become proficient at preparing meals, but as you will see at the end of the chapter, there are meals that are easy to prepare, nutritious and delicious.

Many parents have expressed their struggle with what their teen eats and that it seems that they aren't interested in eating well. One, I believe that is a myth, and two, allowing teens to prepare their own meals or help to prepare the family meals empowers them to be able make healthy meals. This is not something that should be forced, but rather as a way to give teens independence and responsibility.

Rob, a high school senior I worked with, had some obstacles around food. He felt he didn't really know much about food and viewed cooking as something very scary. This was largely due to his family's lifestyle where basically the adults always prepared the meals and were very particular in how they were prepared. In turn, Rob would eat just about anything and would often favor foods that did not have to be cooked or prepared in any way. This steered Rob in the direction of mostly junk food when he was on his own, which was often enough to make it a problem. He reported that he felt sick a lot and said it was starting to get in the way of his social life and even some of the other things he loved to do.

When meeting with Rob and his parents one evening, we started to talk about the idea of Rob learning to prepare food for himself or the family. There was initially some surprise and resistance and Rob's father, in particular, didn't see how this would be helpful. After Rob gave examples of how his lack of confidence and knowledge was impacting his ability to take in good, nutritious foods and ultimately his health and happiness, we went through some suggestions for Rob to get involved with making meals.

We started with something very easy, with Rob working together with his parents to make the first few meals. The first meal we started with was making a fruit salad and then it got more complex, introducing things like smoothies, oatmeal and soups. The more relaxed and confident Rob became around food, the more choices he had. I can't say that Rob totally ditched all processed foods, but there was a major shift. Rob told me that overall he felt better and that his feelings around food and making food became more enjoyable.

Make Your Own Snacks

You can make your own snack foods like potato chips, French fries, popcorn and even pudding in a way that is healthy or at least healthier than what you would get in the store. I will provide some quick recipes at the end of the chapter that are easy to make, nutritious and delicious.

I have had many teens tell me that once they started to make their own snacks or fun food, they felt more in control and found they enjoyed making their own snacks and were surprised by how easy it was. There is nothing wrong with buying healthy or healthier snacks. If you combine that with making your own snacks or fun food, it can be enjoyable and healthy.

I want to make sure that I am being clear. I'm not saying you should snack if you don't want to. You don't have to snack. In fact, some experts would recommend not snacking at all if you are eating three nutrient-dense meals per day and suggest you wouldn't need to snack if you were getting enough nutrients. However, I have found that snacking can be healthy so long as it's done most often with whole, nutrient-dense foods and is not overdone.

One of my favorite healthy snacks is popcorn with Celtic sea salt or Himalayan pink salt and a little olive oil or melted coconut oil. You can also add other seasonings to your liking.

Grow Food

So you want me to be a farmer now? Where would I grow this food anyway? Of course I do not expect everyone to become a farmer or to be able to grow all the food they will ever need. What I can say is that no matter where you live, you can grow something that is edible, even if it's an herb to season your food with such as parsley. There are also ways to grow food using community space, such as a community or school garden. You can also help a neighbor maintain their garden. There are so many inspiring examples of growing food in   seemingly unlikely places, but a few of my favorites are www.urbanfarming.org, www.downtoearth.org and www.sustainabletable.org/251/innovative-agriculture. I have grown food in many areas that would seem out of the ordinary, like indoors. It's just a matter of making use of space.

Many teens enjoy growing food, especially when there are innovative ways to do it. Growing food also has the added benefit of reducing stress and helping teens become more centered and grounded and overall more connected with their food. These benefits are the same for adults.

There is also a satisfaction and comfort in knowing that you grew a portion of your food no matter the size. This is one area I wish we could all have more time to do, as I have watched as this has been a major catalyst in teen health and happiness. I know that when I have worked with teens in group settings and we grew food as a group, the effects were amazing. I do believe there is something about being connected with the soil; whether you are growing food in an open field, the top of a roof, your back deck or your windowsill.

Listen To Your Body/Food Sensitivities

When your body craves a certain food, it is trying to tell you something. Our bodies are hardwired to crave sugar, salt and fat, all things we need in small amounts, but in large quantities, and especially in the case of sugar, are not good for us. So when we do consume sugar, salt and fat, our bodies emit a pleasure response. Food companies and fast food chains understand this concept very well and make sure their 'foods' are loaded with all three, which makes the 'food' they create highly addictive. One of the ways to work with our body's natural desire for sugar, salt and fat is to eat whole, nutrient-dense foods.

So should we listen to our bodies? Yes, and consider what our bodies might be missing when we crave sugar, salt or fat. Many experts agree that when we crave sweets, it is often a sign of dehydration and is a signal that our body wants glucose. It also can be a sign that we need more high-quality protein in our diet.

One of the best ways to satisfy this craving is to add sweet cooked vegetables, such as carrots, sweet potatoes and/or onions, to our meals. Another way to satisfy sugar cravings is to eat fruit. It will provide you with healthy natural glucose and in most cases will also provide you with water. It is beneficial to eat a handful of nuts or seeds with your fruit, as it helps to keep your blood sugar from spiking and provides you with sustained energy.

When we are craving salty foods, that's usually an indication that our body is missing the minerals in salt, especially sodium. The thing is, most table salt is very often stripped of its nutrients due to processing. I recommend using Celtic sea salt, Himalayan pink salt or consuming pumpkin seeds and/or sunflower seeds instead of using table salt.

When your body craves fats or fried foods, it wants a good healthy source of fat. If you find that you are craving fats or fried foods, it's usually a sign that you are not getting enough good fat in your diet. A great way to take in good fats is to eat an avocado or have a few almonds.

It's important to listen to our bodies when it comes to being sensitive or even allergic to certain foods. Sensitivities and allergies to foods can range from mild to severe, to the point where they can be life-threatening. In the severe and life-threatening instances, there are pretty clear signs there that you have to pay attention to. When the sensitivities and allergies are on the mild side, it can be harder to recognize. This is where a food journal really comes in handy, although, you don't need to have a food journal to notice how certain foods make you feel.

One of the easiest ways to find out whether you have a sensitivity or an allergy to certain foods is to leave them out of your diet for a week, then

44

slowly add them back in one at a time over several days. You would want to do this with individual foods. For instance, you wouldn't want to cut out apples, bread and cheese from your diet then add them all back in on the same day, because if you did have some sort of reaction, you wouldn't know which of the three you are reacting to. Add one in, see if you have any type of reaction, then take it out the next day, and add the next food in and continue until you have gone through all of the foods that you were suspicious of.

Another important point is that sometimes we develop sensitivities or allergies to certain foods over time. I know some teens have expressed surprise that they were allergic to a certain food when they had no indication that they were allergic as a child.

One of the symptoms Allison was dealing with when she came to me was severe headaches. They would often be so debilitating that she would have to stay in bed for days. Allison had been to see her family physician, who had run many tests but was still unsure what was causing them. However, her physician was starting to suspect a food allergy. Eventually, we discovered that her allergy wasn't so much to a particular food as it was to the red dyes often used in these 'foods'. Once we knew that the dyes were the issue, Allison was again able to enjoy most foods so long as she avoided the ones that contained red dyes.

Start Small

Perhaps one of the best recommendations I can share with regard to nutrition from my work with teens is to start small. You do not have to make major changes all at once. The changes should be made in a way that will work and is sustainable. A lot of times this looks like introducing healthier versions of foods one at a time, a little at a time.

Richie loved to eat breakfast bars that where highly processed and loaded with sugar, dyes and other additives. "I think I am addicted to them. I sometimes have eight in a day." Once we determined that Richie wanted to change this habit, we came up with a plan that included starting to replace these bars with apples and almonds, which would give him the sweets and good fats he craved.

We realized that having Richie go from eight of these bars a day to none probably wouldn't work or be sustainable. What we agreed on is that we would replace one of Richie's breakfasts bars with either a half or a whole apple and a few almonds. We did this for ten days before substituting more fruits and nuts for the breakfast bars. Over a period of about six months, Richie was down to one bar a day and sometimes not even that. He was amazed to find that eating fruits and nuts kept him full and also satisfied his need for sweets and fats. The amount of fruits and nuts he needed began to diminish as well.

You don't always need to start with something that you consume that much of every day; you can start with something you have only once a day or a few times per week. The idea is to start with one change then add in other areas you would like to change. I don't want to discourage anyone who wants to dive into making as many healthy changes as possible in a short amount of time. Indeed, there are times when that is what is needed. Remember, you want the changes to stick and become a way of life; you don't want to add in any undue pressure or stress. Stress can lead right back to unhealthy habits that can impact teen health and happiness.

You may notice that as you start with small changes, making additional changes becomes easier and will stick. So have fun and give yourself the time you need to succeed.

Give Yourself A Break/Get Back On Track

We are all human and sometimes we are going to eat or drink something that isn't good for us. You may even have a 'bad' few days, week or weeks. The key is to give yourself a break and don't beat yourself up. Get back on track. And that may mean you need to start slowly again.

What I've found is that striving to make healthier choices 90% of the time is a good target to aim for. Of course, 100% is better. In most teenagers' lives, 90% of the time is more realistic and also gives them freedom to enjoy the so-called spoils of the teen years like pizza and ice cream. No, I am not suggesting that this is something that should happen often. Remember though, you can actually make a healthier version of pizza and ice cream. There are even healthier versions of soda.

If for some reason things have gone off track, just get back on no matter how long it's been. There is no rule that states you can be off track for so long before getting back on. I know that some teens and their families figured that since they were off the track for so long, it didn't matter if that got back on. Yes, it matters. Get back on, give yourself a break and be healthy and happy.

If you are a teen reading this book, you can ultimately make your own choices. Some teens I have worked with felt at the mercy of their parents or guardians, even when they have asked to make changes. Most teens, especially when on the younger side, are not the ones buying the food. There is a choice here also. The choice is to ask to get involved in helping to shop for food. Asking to help prepare food is also a way you can make choices. You can also choose not to drink that soda or sugary drink every day. You would be hard pressed to find an adult who would force you to drink soda rather than water. You can decide not to eat fast food and opt for the healthier version. You can even decide to grow a garden.

If you're an adult reading this book, you do have choices when it comes to helping teens have better nutrition. Ultimately, teens are going to look to you to lead by example; it's not what you say, but what you do that's important. I always say to adults that if you don't want to make these changes yourself, at the very least don't get in the way of your teen/s making these changes. Support the teens in your life and show them your support by helping them get what they need.

RECIPES

The following are recipes that I know have been used by the teens I have worked with. They are all meatless recipes; however, you can add in meat to the recipes if you so choose.

If you're a teen reading this book and want to try making these recipes yourself but haven't had much experience with preparing food before, please ask for help. There's no need to get the fire department in on your food preparation. As always, I recommend using organic, whole-food ingredients when possible.

Fun Foods/Snacks

Potato Chips

Ingredients:
3 medium or large red potatoes (can substitute purple or sweet potatoes)
2 1/2 Tablespoons olive, avocado or melted coconut oil (can adjust amount, if needed)
Celtic sea or Himalayan pink salt and black pepper, to taste
Other seasonings you may enjoy, such as rosemary or dill (optional)

Preparation:
1. Preheat the oven to 400 *.
2. Lightly grease a baking sheet with coconut oil.
3. Slice potatoes into about 1/8-inch slices and place them in a bowl.
4. Toss the slices with your chosen healthy oil and seasonings of your choice.
5. Place the slices flat and separately on the lightly-greased baking sheet.
6. Bake in the oven until golden brown, approximately 10 to 15 minutes.
7. Season again lightly with your chosen seasoning as soon as they come out of the oven, if needed.
8. Let the potato chips cool before eating.
9. You may store in a container in the refrigerator for up to five days.

* I have a friend who swears by doing this on low broil. You can see if different temperature settings will work best for you.

Please note: You can use essentially the same process to make French fries, simply by cutting the potatoes into French-fry-sized portions. You do not have to season them with oil first, but you can.

Chocolate Avocado Pudding

Ingredients:

2 ripe Hass avocados

1/3 cup Grade B maple syrup or coconut nectar

3 Tablespoons raw cacao powder

1 teaspoon vanilla extract

1/8 teaspoon Celtic sea or Himalayan pink salt

1/8 teaspoon cinnamon

Preparation:

1. Open the avocados with a large knife by carefully cutting them in a circle from top to bottom of the skin, then twist to separate the sides. De-pit the avocado by carefully hitting the blade of the knife into the pit and twisting. This will take the pit out with no fuss.
2. Scoop the avocado out with a spoon (discarding the skin) into your food processor or blender and add the sweetener, raw cacao powder, vanilla extract, sea salt and cinnamon and process until smooth.
3. Once processed, check for taste and adjust with additions of any of the ingredients accordingly.

4. Serve in bowls and optionally top with fresh blueberries, strawberries, shredded coconut or hemp seeds.

Breakfast

Breakfast Smoothie Quickie

Ingredients:

1 ripe Hass avocado and/or 1 Tablespoon raw almond butter

1 to 1 1/2 cups of unsweetened nondairy milk (almond, coconut, hemp)

1 whole green apple, cut into four sections

2 teaspoons raw cacao powder and/or 1 Tablespoon of vanilla extract

1 handful of baby spinach

1/2 cup fresh or frozen berries of your choice

Preparation:

1. Add the avocado/almond butter, green apple, raw cacao powder/vanilla extract, baby spinach and berries of your choice to a blender or food processor.
2. Add the 1 to 1 1/2 cups of nondairy milk and process until smooth.
3. May be eaten right away or stored in a glass container to be eaten at another meal.

Mixed Vegetable Wraps

Ingredients:

4 whole-grain or gluten-free tortillas wraps

1/2 cup tomatoes, chopped

1 avocado, diced, or you can stir into a spread, if preferred

1 cup of celery or carrots, chopped

1/2 cup black olives, chopped

1 leaf of red leaf lettuce per tortilla (you can substitute or add spinach if you prefer)

1/2 teaspoon Celtic sea or Himalayan pink salt

Other seasonings, if desired (optional)

Preparation:

1. Lay each tortilla flat and put one leaf of red leaf lettuce on each tortilla.
2. In a bowl, combine the tomatoes, avocado, celery/carrots, black olives, sea salt and any other seasonings you desire and mix thoroughly.
3. Spread the mixture evenly across each piece of red leaf lettuce on tortilla.
4. Roll up tortilla and enjoy.

Please note: I always opt for a bit less in the tortillas so that they roll and stay together nicely. This is a pretty easy recipe to experiment with so get creative. I sometimes use shredded red cabbage or romaine lettuce instead of the red leaf lettuce and I have fun switching up the vegetables to include red bell peppers, cucumbers, sugar snap peas and/or green beans.

Dinner

Roasted Butternut Squash

Ingredients:

1 large butternut squash, seeds removed and cut in half (can roast seeds separately, if desired)

3 Tablespoons melted coconut or olive oil

1/2 teaspoon black pepper

1/2 teaspoon Celtic sea or Himalayan pink salt

Clean filtered/spring water

Preparation:

1. Preheat oven to 425 degrees.

2. Carefully cut the squash in half lengthwise (they are usually hard to cut so be extra careful).

3. Scoop the seeds out of the squash and set aside if you want to roast them or discard if you do not.

4. Mix together the coconut oil or olive oil, black pepper and sea salt, rub the oil mixture on the outside of the squash and carefully poke holes in the skin with a sharp knife.

5. Next, place the butternut squash face down (skin side up) in a shallow baking dish with a tiny bit of water and roast for 45 to 50 minutes or until tender.

6. Turn over with the skin side down and cook until tender, approximately 10 to 15 additional minutes.

7. Serve as-is or cut it up into smaller chunks.

8. Can top with grass-fed cultured butter, a little Grade B maple syrup or drizzle with coconut amino acids.

Suggestions:

- I always wait until I can poke a knife through both sides to serve.
- You can roast the seeds in a separate pan with coconut oil and sea salt. They make a delicious and nutritious snack.
- When making the seeds, roast until they are golden brown and crunchy. You can season any way you like. My favorite is with a little olive oil and sea salt.

Chapter Four

Movement & Exercise

Sitting is the new smoking. What does that mean? The idea is that too much sitting is just as bad for your health or worse for your health than smoking. To be clear, smoking isn't good for you either. Some of the effects of prolonged sitting are an increased risk of cancer, heart disease, obesity, muscular issues, depression and diabetes. These are some of the many reasons why exercise and movement are so vital to health and happiness.

Our bodies are designed, want and need to move. When we don't, it goes against our natural inclinations. Movement can take many forms and I don't think there is really any one form of movement that is superior to another. Exercise is generally an activity that we carry out to improve health. It can be a part of movement, but it isn't always necessarily the same thing.

There are many ways to move and exercise and the benefits of movement and exercise to health and happiness are plentiful. A few benefits are that exercise helps maintain a healthy weight, it builds muscle mass and also helps maintain strong, flexible muscles. It increases your metabolism and the efficiency of moving nutrients throughout your body and it helps to reduce stress and improves your mood by increasing the level of endorphins in your bloodstream, which are responsible for feelings of happiness and joy. Exercise also boosts serotonin, which helps us to feel calm and centered, gives a boost to our immune system and helps to improve brainpower and capacity to learn.

While we make the distinction between exercise and movement, both movement and exercise help with learning, thinking and creativity. Exercise also gives us more energy and promotes deeper and more restful sleep. Exercise can and should be fun. This doesn't mean there isn't work and effort involved; it means that there are ways to exercise that don't have to be something we dread.

I am often asked by teens and their parents which is the best form of exercise. In my experience with teens, I have found that as long as they are moving their body in some fashion every day in a way that requires an output of energy and effort that increases strength, blood flow, cardiovascular capacity and flexibility, it doesn't really matter. The most common thread that I found throughout is that any form of movement or exercise has to be sustainable and enjoyable. I have worked with teens whose favorite thing to do was to take a long walk and others who found that playing soccer was something they loved.

There are many ways to move and exercise. I go through a few here, not to try to persuade anyone to adopt one form of movement or exercise, yet to offer what I have found to work for teen health and happiness. I do not attempt to include all the great forms of exercise here, so if something you enjoy does not appear here, it doesn't mean you should stop.

A mixture of strength or resistance training, cardiovascular training and flexibility training is generally a good balance to strive for. I always recommend warming up for between 5 to 10 minutes before starting any form of exercise.

Cardiovascular Training

Cardiovascular training, sometimes referred to as cardio or aerobic training, depends on the use of oxygen for energy. Cardio training helps build the efficient use of oxygen. Walking, running, hiking, biking, swimming, rowing, cross-country skiing, jumping rope, dancing and aerobics are some of the best but not the only forms of cardiovascular training.

For optimal cardiovascular training, many experts suggest calculating a target heart rate and keeping it at that rate for at least 10 minutes. I also recommend getting to know yourself well and working within a heart rate; however, don't let calculating a heart rate stop you from cardiovascular training.

A cautionary note is that some of these activities, like walking, hiking and biking, if done too leisurely, while having other benefits, will not have much cardiovascular benefit. For teens, it's about finding something that works for them and will have the benefits of cardiovascular training.

Like always, you want to start slowly if you have been inactive for a long time or never really exercised, then you can move to bigger challenges. Try running or any cardio activity for 10 to 15 minutes the first week, then add on three to five minutes each week until you increase to 30 minutes or more. This does not have to happen every single day. Four to five days a week is a good amount to strive for. If that's not possible, there is benefit to even one day per week.

Flexibility/Balance Training

Flexibility training generally helps one increase their range of motion or flexibility. Flexibility training can improve posture, increase range of motion of muscles and joints, prevent injuries, increase blood to muscles and joints and it generally feels good to stretch. Stretching, yoga, Pilates, martial arts and activities that use range of motion will all increase flexibility. Many of these activities have benefits beyond just increasing flexibility like stress reduction and increased strength.

Balance training helps with building balance and also body awareness or knowing where your body is in a given space. Balance training will help improve your agility, strength, body awareness, coordination and stability, to name a few of its benefits.

There doesn't seem to be a set amount of time to spend with flexibility or balance training to get the benefits; however, in general, the more time spent, the better the results.

Strength & Resistance Training

This type of training uses some type of resistance — e.g., weights, bands, body weight, etc. — that generally targets a specific or large group of muscles in order to build strength, endurance and tone muscles. Taking time to engage in strength training will help prevent injury, increase bone density, maintain weight, tone muscles, increase strength and may increase an overall feeling of confidence.

There are a variety of strength-training exercises, and as explained above, some use weights, resistance bands and/or body weight. Some of my favorites that do not require any equipment are pushups, sit-ups, planks (planking) and hip extensions. And of course, using weights, resistance bands or other equipment to provide resistance are great ways to build strength and get the benefits of strength and resistance training.

As with flexibility and balance, there doesn't seem to be a set amount of time needed to be spent, but in this case, it's more about the amount of repetitions or amount of resistance. That being said, doing pushups for 30 seconds, while providing some benefit, may not be quite long enough.

There are some major categories of exercise or movement that incorporate cardiovascular, strength, flexibility and balance training in them. I discuss a few below that I have had success with and that, in my experience, teens enjoy and benefit from.

Sports

There are a variety of sports one could participate in and to go into detail about every single one of them would be a whole book unto itself. There is also some debate as to what can be considered a sport. I have found that it matters little and that there really isn't one that is superior to any other. As mentioned above, it should be enjoyable and sustainable.

I am going to keep my definition of a sport pretty simply: A sport is an activity that requires movement, effort, physical as well as mental training and generally involves competition against a team or an individual. I have had those who argue with me that the card game of poker or the game of darts is a sport. While I respect the effort that goes into becoming a well-versed poker or dart player (I love to play darts), I think arguing for its status as a sport misses the point in this context.

Some do not like the competition aspect of sports and that's okay. While sports can be a great way to exercise, move, learn about teamwork and how to handle success and failure, they are not the only way to exercise and move. I have had many teens tell me that they just aren't into sports and that's why they don't exercise. I think sometimes exercise and movement get confused with sports. You don't have to like sports to do pushups or go for a walk.

Martial Arts

Martial arts are oftentimes defined as some sort of combat or fighting discipline and are considered to be a sport by many. However, martial arts can be so much more; having spiritual, physical and healing components to them. Oftentimes, martial arts are viewed more as a way of life than just a form of exercise or movement.

There are many wonderful forms of martial arts and to go into all of them in detail is outside the scope of this book. What I can say is that the ones I am fond of are the ones I have studied myself or have watched teens enjoy, so the following is in no way meant to exclude any form of martial arts.

Most forms of martial arts will have cardio, strength, flexibility and balance training incorporated into the practice to some degree. Two of my favorites are Aikido and Tai Chi. While considered by some to be somewhat less physical forms of martial arts, I have found them both to be physically challenging coupled with a spiritual or way-of-life component that is hard to separate.

It doesn't matter so much what form or style of martial arts one chooses to practice, what does seem to matter is who the instructor is, the philosophy of the school or dojo and how comfortable one is with what is being taught.

Yoga, undoubtedly, has a spiritual and some might even say a religious component to it. This seems to depend, like marital arts, on which instructor or school one goes to. Yoga is a discipline that combines breathing techniques, meditation and a wide range of body postures that also vary in difficulty. In general, one builds up to the more complex postures through a series of less complex postures.

Some would say that yoga has less of a cardiovascular component than it does strength, balance and flexibility. Be that as it may, there is still a cardiovascular component to it, and much like marital arts, yoga has the additional benefits of stress reduction and mindfulness.

In recent years, there has been an explosion of yoga studios and instructors. While many are wonderful and reputable, there are also those that have not put in enough time to be able to teach the discipline safely and effectively. There are even programs where one can become a yoga instructor in as short as a weekend or a couple of months. Although this may be fine and the instructor may indeed be a good one, I recommend doing some research before taking any classes.

Movement, How Is It Different?

Exercise and movement are not always the same. Taking the definition of exercise above, not all movement would be considered exercise. Movement is simply that, movement, and I recommend moving as often as possible. This is not to say move in a way that is disruptive or destructive, but to move so that you can get blood flowing, your brain moving and just give your body a chance to be in a different position, as it doesn't matter a whole lot what kind of movement it is.

So What Do We Do Now?

'I know that exercise is good for me, but I feel like I move around enough so I don't have to exercise.' This is something I hear from teens regularly. I think, again, sometimes there is confusion about what exercise is and isn't. The interesting thing is that I hear this from teens that are both very active and not very active. What I have found is that a lot depends on lifestyle; meaning that if exercise/movement are built into daily life or viewed as a part of it, then it is easier to maintain. It often is a matter of just getting started if you haven't already.

As we did in the previous chapter, a good place to start is with the questions below. In case you aren't reading this book chapter by chapter, I will provide some suggestions about how to approach answering these questions.

These questions are not about a right or wrong answer. Don't worry about what you think the answers are supposed to be; just answer as honestly as you can. It's about bringing awareness to what is happening and having time for reflection. You may find that just answering these questions provides new insight or a new perspective.

So whether you're a teen or adult reading this book, the questions are here to get you to think about your exercise and movement habits and what they look like. If you're an adult that isn't a parent to teens but works with teens, answer the questions based on what you have observed from working with teens.

As with all the questions in this book, grab a piece of paper and a pen, get comfortable, sit back, relax and have fun answering the following questions:

- *Question 1:* What is/are the teen/s in your life's amount of exercise and movement like? As with the nutrition exercise, it may be helpful to write down or map out what a typical day looks like.
- *Question 2:* Overall, is/are the teen/s in your life getting enough exercise?
- *Question 3:* What types of exercise or movement does/do the teen/s in your life seem to enjoy?
- *Question 4:* What does the teen's/s' general attitude towards exercise and movement seem to be? Is it something to be avoided, a chore, enjoyable? Do they look forward to it?
- *Question 5:* What are the biggest challenges to the teen/s in your life enjoying more exercise or movement?

As with all the questions in this book, I suggest revisiting these questions from time to time to note any changes and to see your progress. I offer the following recommendations based on my work with teens in the field that will help with the answers to the above questions.

Again, this is not meant to be comprehensive, but rather a glimpse into how exercise and movement can help teens be happy and healthy. I also provide some examples of how these recommendations have been and are being used. It would be impossible to go through every scenario or share every experience I have had; however, these provide some examples and help with motivating teens to exercise and move.

Recommendations/Examples

Keep It Simple

I made the same recommendation in Chapter Three on nutrition and I believe that this is a good rule of thumb for many of the recommendations throughout this book.

Many times I have watched a teen and/or their family try to make too many changes too soon or be too overreaching. Not only can this cause injury, it is hard to sustain. It won't do much good if suddenly the preferred method of exercise costs a lot of money or requires a long drive to get to or long hours that cannot be sustained. Of course, if you feel you can sustain these types of commitments, then by all means, do so. The point here is that you need not make a huge commitment right away. I know some who have argued this point with me saying that you need to be all in and commit to something for it to work. Quite honestly, I have seen that work as well, though it doesn't have to be a zero-to-one-hundred proposition.

I remember working with a small group of teens in a setting where they were not encouraged to move or exercise. They weren't prevented from doing so, it's just that they weren't encouraged or readily given the means to. This led to weight gain, mild depression, lack of strength or muscle tone for most and left the group feeling lethargic.

We started by talking a 10-minute walk for a week, then we added in sit-ups, pushups and some basic stretches. In some cases, we started with one sit-up and one pushup until we could increase the amount. Since many of the teens in this group had not been active in a while, we kept things pretty simple and only got more complex when they were ready or wanted to challenge themselves.

After only the first 10 days, I noticed that the group seemed a little more lively and energetic. Most of the teens said they felt a little sore but liked how they felt. As the weeks passed, some in the group were setting goals for themselves and wanted to make sure that they kept exercising and moving. They also said that they realized they didn't need much to exercise. At the end of my time with this group, they seemed happy, as one of them said, "I feel different; better. I am not so down. I look forward to exercising."

Not everyone is going to love to exercise and love movement, but at the very least they can enjoy it to some degree. They key is to start small.

Set Realistic Goals

If a teen has been mostly sedentary for a while, then we cannot expect him or her to run a marathon after a few weeks of being active. Of course, teens in general can achieve strength, flexibility and cardiovascular fitness more quickly than adults can after being inactive. As in the example I gave above, beginning with basic movements and exercises can be a good place to start. As we know, everyone is a unique individual and the goals can be individualized for each teen. The idea is to set teens up for success.

Teens should be setting their own goals, and of course, adults can support and help them in doing so. Not only will this empower and motivate them, the goals will ultimately be better and more sustainable since they know themselves best.

Exercise should be fun and interesting. It doesn't have to fall into a mundane routine. While, of course, it is best to combine strength, flexibility and cardiovascular training daily, you don't have to do all three every day. In fact, there should be rest incorporated into your routine. This doesn't mean no movement at all, but a one-day break from exercise to give the body time to recover.

Different activities can be mixed up that provide exercise during the year. For instance, running is a great way to build cardiovascular fitness and you can substitute a different type of cardiovascular activity, such as cross-country skiing, in the winter. I also recommend trying different kinds of sports. The latest trend is for teens and even preteens to specialize in one sport in the hopes of gaining experience and honing skills on a higher level. This leads to another trend, overuse injuries, which are happening earlier and earlier.

Let It Be Their Choice

Far too often I have watched adults push teens into physical activities they do not want to do. It's understandable that adults want the teens in their lives to share in an activity or sport that the adults themselves love. However, many of the teens I have worked with felt an enormous amount of pressure from adults to like or participate in certain types of activities or sports.

To be clear, I am not saying that there aren't times when caring adults need to intervene and make suggestions when a teen's health and happiness is at stake. What I am saying is that forcing teens — or really anyone for that matter — to participate in an activity usually backfires. At best, the teen will tolerate it until they don't have to do it anymore; at worst, it causes resentment and strained relationships. Also worth mentioning is that oftentimes teens will avoid having anything to do with that activity once they are finished with it.

I have worked with families where they came to an agreement that the teen would try an activity for six months to a year or, when relevant, a sports season. At the end of this time, they could decide if they wanted to continue or not. This can certainly work and can be a compromise.

A final note on this is that I have watched overzealous parents turn their teens completely off from sports or physical activity because they were so gung-ho at the games and practices. I have witnessed some troubling behavior by adults at games and practices where they have way overstepped their bounds on various levels. This never ends well and causes multiple issues. Unfortunately, these poor examples set by parents, family members, coaches, etc., are becoming more common.

The good news is that most teens will show an affinity for certain types of exercise or movement and will likely approach the adults in their lives for support. When they don't or if exercise of any kind seems not to be their thing, approaching this as a partnership for their health and happiness is the way to go.

Move Every Hour

This does not mean you should exercise every hour. It means you should get up, move around or change your position at least every hour. Unfortunately, today's teens have many devices, activities and forms of entertainment that encourage them to sit for long periods of time, including how most spend their school day (I will talk about this much more in the chapter on learning and creativity).

It does not matter much how you are moving, only that you are. There are many great stretching techniques you can do after sitting for a long period of time. If you are not able to get up and move every hour, then try stretching in your seat. It's as easy as planting your feet firmly on the ground and reaching your arms above your head as high as you can without your feet coming off the ground. I also recommend that if you can perform the same task with the same level of quality standing that you can while sitting, then stand. There are many great standing workstations, desks, etc., that work well in this situation.

I remember working with Alex, who was fascinated with all things technological. He was particularly good at writing code for websites and started his own business at age 16. Alex, his parents and I were concerned with the fact that Alex would spend long hours sitting and wasn't getting the benefits of moving. While Alex was smart and likable, he was starting to show signs of mild depression, and overall, he didn't look — or judging from his own words — feel healthy. "I like how I spend my time. I enjoy it. I should probably move around a little more. I just get so focused on what I am doing."

This presented a very real conflict for me. The educator/creator side of me wanted to not interrupt the flow of his work; the health coach/holistic practitioner side of me wanted to make sure he was moving. I also knew that he didn't have to stop thinking or his flow in order to move; in fact, movement, creativity and learning all go together.

What we did for Alex is have him set a reminder alarm on one of his devices that would remind to him to move. We generally only used this when he was at home or outside of school. Since Alex had portable technology, he didn't have to stop what he was doing in order to move. We did build in a safety where he used sticky notes and/or a small white board just in case for some reason he didn't have his portable technology with him and wanted to remember to move without them. I think Alex was surprised to find that he rather enjoyed moving about while he was thinking or writing code. As it turns out, Alex was moving a lot — more than every hour — and it seemed to give him more creative energy.

Moving is not separate from thinking, learning and working. We need to get away from the notion that if you are moving, you're not being productive or that moving like that is for children. It isn't.

Chapter Five

Spiritual Health

What is Spirituality? Spirituality is a belief in a purpose higher than yourself or something that transcends your heart and soul. Spirituality does not necessarily mean one follows a certain religious doctrine or set of beliefs, though it could. Spirituality touches our soul. It feels human and pure and allows us to feel connected with each other and everything around us in some way. It doesn't have to be attached to a particular religion.

Spirituality often gets confused with religion. Religion and spirituality are not inherently separate, nor are they quite the same. You can be spiritual without following a particular religion, much the same way you can be religious but not at all spiritual. I am sure we have all heard and experienced many instances where folks who proclaim themselves to be morally superior because they follow a particular religion have perpetrated acts against humanity that are horrific.

Any spiritual or religious teaching that proclaims they have found the exact right way for anyone to live is flawed, not only on an intellectual level, but on a spiritual and social level as well. Religion certainly has its place and that place is not to divide the world into believers and nonbelievers and the beliefs, rituals and practices of others into righteous and nonrighteous. I believe its place is to provide a connection to our humanity and everything that makes us human.

Spirituality is a different matter entirely. When viewed as a belief in a purpose higher than yourself, it takes on a different meaning and looks and feels different in practice. I know that in my work with teens we talk about

70

how spiritual health or spirituality many times conjures up images of someone meditating, sitting in a yoga pose or hugging a tree. Of course, any of these can be part of spiritual health or practice, as spirituality is complex and can take different forms. Here in the West, talking about spirituality or even mentioning the word is often equated with being a hippie, Buddhist monk or tree hugger. It's not always something teens are used to talking about and they may not have thought about it much or had the opportunity to talk about it.

The thing is that spiritual health is equally as important as any other area of health. If the spirit is sick, it leads to many imbalances, which may ultimately have a negative impact on teen health and happiness. There are clear signs and symptoms that manifest when spiritual health is out of balance, such as depression or lack of joy, addictions, not being able to connect emotionally, apathy, depersonalization and a propensity towards suicide.

Teens in our society are in many ways cut off from their spirituality. In a lot of settings, any talk or notion of spirituality is discouraged. For example, most teens spend their weekdays in school, which systematically disconnects and disengages them from their spirituality, mainly because the opportunities to engage and connect aren't seized and are pushed aside in favor of 'the standards' or are steered clear of for fear of deviating from the 'curriculum'. This happens in schools that have a religious affiliation as well and sometimes even more so.

Looking at examples, such as the practice of Tai Chi, are helpful in getting a different perspective on spirituality. Many of you have probably at least heard of this practice and may think it is simply a way to maintain health. Another dimension of this practice is the belief in 'chi', which is an inner energy that flows throughout the body. When this is out of balance or blocked, this can cause disease.

There is also the idea of balance and harmony. While this may not be overtly spiritual on the surface, it is a philosophy that believes in the power of our inner strength and the ability to heal ourselves. This has a strong resemblance to what many believe is the balance of nature; how life has the ability to heal itself, how if this balance is upset, the effects will be noticeable. I would argue that when one practices organic gardening, ecologically-friendly behaviors, respecting other creatures' habitats and needs, using the principles of balance and nature's way of growing and providing, this is spiritual in that it is a belief in a purpose higher than ourselves.

There is much research from many specialty areas, such as social psychology, that we, as human beings, are healthier and happier and even more intellectually aroused when we are part of something higher than ourselves. A common theme when I work with teens is that they feel there is something missing in their lives. They feel this because they know deep down that there is something more; something is missing. Their spirituality is not being fed. In most cases, it is being beaten down or worse, distinctly and particularly guided in such a way as to remove any true reflection. Most teens know this deep down, even if they can't always articulate it. This causes angst and a deep unrest that sometimes is hard to uncover, which means that it is much more important to do the work in this area.

I can say that the unbalance in teen spiritual health often does stem from the adults that teens are surrounded by. No, I am not saying that adults are purposefully making teens spiritually unhealthy. What I am saying is that when the adults teens are surrounded by are spiritually unhealthy, it throws teens out of balance because they do not have an example to follow.

For teens, a reflection on their spirituality isn't something they come across naturally. Usually, they have to seek it out or come across it on their own. Of course, many families do have a spiritual practice or at least a way to reflect on spirituality and this can be very helpful. It's not hard to be thrown off balance spiritually, especially for teens with all they have coming at them, along with the hormonal and other changes they are going through.

While below in the recommendations section I do talk about meditation in order to be spiritual, you don't necessarily have to meditate. I think spirituality is more than just one thing. In the end, it is a way of being more than it is a practice or way of thinking.

There is drastically little, if any, thought given to the spiritual aspect of teenagers, perhaps because many are afraid to cross this boundary, thinking it's too far of an overreach. I do think there are ways to have conversations and action around spirituality. The questions arise about how to define spirituality and who gets to do so. I provided a definition above that I believe is workable in the context of this book. In no way is it meant to be the end of the conversation on what spirituality is.

In this chapter I go right into the questions, recommendations and examples, since they will provide enough of a framework to understand the dynamics of spirituality.

So What Do We Do Now?

Where do we go from here? Spirituality, as we know, is complex and overlooked in teen health and happiness. The first place we can go is to start a dialog with teens about spirituality and to be open to exploring this further. If we start with the premise that we are connected to something higher than ourselves or just pose this idea as a question, it can be a way to further exploration and exploration it must be. Are we connected to something higher than ourselves? No matter your answer, how do you know?

We need to be careful not to indoctrinate teens to one way of thinking or believing. But wait, you just said spirituality is a belief in a purpose higher than ourselves or something that transcends our hearts and souls. Isn't that indoctrination? It could be if it is used as a way to confine thinking or action. Where spirituality gets tricky is that there are many ways to look at it. Some would say riding their motorcycle is a spiritual experience for them. I wholeheartedly believe that it is, as I do with many other experiences. It's when we start describing what the experience was like that we can uncover the spiritual component.

In my work with teens, a spiritual experience can be hard to describe but almost always includes words like heart, soul, flow, faith, connection, joy, happy and/or peaceful. Some teens have described it as knowing everything was going to be okay and knowing that they are not alone. Oscar, a high school sophomore, described it to me in this way: "Sometimes when I'm just sitting and thinking, or I could be walking too, I feel in my heart that everything is okay. I sorta think that everything around me is okay too, like there's this little stuff that doesn't matter as much as I thought it did."

I believe this is a spiritual experience because something was happening at a level that goes beyond thinking and goes more to a place of feeling. Some may call this simple emotion, and since we know teens can have intense and rapidly-changing emotions, it's nothing more than that. I disagree. While emotion can be part of a spiritual experience, that feeling

74

that Oscar described of everything around him being okay is something more than just emotion.

As we did in the previous chapters, a good place to start is with the questions below. In case you aren't reading this book chapter by chapter, I will provide some suggestions about how to approach answering these questions.

These questions are not about a right or wrong answer. Don't worry about what you think the answers are supposed to be; just answer as honestly as you can. It's about bringing awareness to what is happening and having time for reflection. You may find that just answering these questions provides new insight or a new perspective.

So whether you're a teen or adult reading this book, the questions are here to get you to think about spiritual health habits and what they look like. If you're an adult that isn't a parent to teens but works with teens, answer the questions based on what you have observed from working with teens.

As with all the questions in this book, grab a piece of paper and a pen, get comfortable, sit back, relax and have fun answering the following questions:

- *Question 1:* Have you ever had a conversation with the teen/s in your life about spirituality or anything resembling spirituality? If you have, what was the conversation like?
- *Question 2:* Does/do the teen/s in your life have a regular spiritual practice (something that you think is spiritual)? What does it look like?
- *Question 3:* Are there any spiritual practices that you think the teen/s in your life would enjoy? What are they?

- *Question 4:* What is/are the teen/s in your life's general feeling towards spirituality?

- *Question 5:* What are the biggest challenges to the teen/s in your life having spiritual health?

    As with all the questions in this book, I suggest revisiting these questions from time to time to note any changes and to see your progress. These questions are a guide to exploration and I invite you to come up with your own.

    I offer the following recommendations based on my work with teens in the field that will offer some insight into the above questions.

Recommendations/Examples

Start The Dialog

    So many of the teens I have worked with have expressed their appreciation when adults dialog with them about spiritual health. Dialog is about people freely expressing their views, and when teens can do this with each other and adults around spirituality, the experience can be very rich.

    A great way to start a dialog is to ask questions. You can start with the questions outlined above, use your own or some combination of the two. A question I have had success with is, what is spirituality? From there, follow-up questions can be asked. It's important to remain open and allow the dialog to unfold, not trying to push it in one direction or another. It is worth repeating that spirituality does not necessarily mean religion and that any dialog on spirituality should never be only about one set of beliefs.

I know that adults who work with teens are sometimes apprehensive about starting a dialog on spirituality. They fear that this may go outside the bounds of what their work with teens entails. You must absolutely adhere to the guidelines of your work, so if having this dialog goes beyond those guidelines, I recommend creating the space for this dialog to happen amongst the teens.

Working in therapeutic environments with teens — some that were overt about spirituality and some that weren't — spirituality on some level would emerge. Some of the dialog and work around it can be intense, as spirituality is intensely personal. When the dialog is really about having a dialog and giving everyone equal opportunity to express their views, it generally works well.

For example, with a group of teens I worked with, we would come together to dialog about spirituality. We did this more on an as-it-arose basis, so it wasn't forced. I was careful not to have any preconceived outcomes, as I wanted the dialog to evolve naturally on its own. A way to do this is to be transparent about it from the start and have every member of the group set agreements for how the dialog will go. I won't provide a list of shoulds or shouldn'ts, as I think it is best for those to emerge from the group itself.

An important point to note is that as an adult you don't have to be the one to start the dialog, but rather, as mentioned above, create the space for it to happen. Oftentimes, with the groups of teens I've worked with the dialog would happen amongst the teens without me being involved. It doesn't matter much how the dialog comes about, so long as it's happening. Some may argue that there should always be an adult present when dialog of this nature happens. First, I think this is unrealistic, and second, if dialog on spirituality is supposed to become a part of teens' lives, they must be allowed to actually have that dialog.

Seize Opportunities

It's also important to seize the opportunities to dialog about or practice spirituality. At first, it may seem like these opportunities are few and far between. This has not been my experience. My experience in spending a great deal of time with teens is that these opportunities are plentiful.

There are so many experiences that teens have, especially in today's fast-paced, technologically-based world, but few are totally devoid of some spiritual aspect. The current state of the world is rife with opportunities to dialog on a purpose higher than ourselves or experiences that transcend our hearts and souls. One example might be, at the time of the writing of this book, the United States is in the midst of a hotly-contested presidential campaign where one candidate is seemingly stirring up issues of morality and justice. This does not necessarily mean that any dialog on this automatically is or has to be spiritual. I would be surprised if a dialog on the current U.S. Presidential Election or any election worldwide did not bring up aspects of spirituality.

When I say 'seize the opportunity,' I don't mean force the issue or be waiting to pounce on anything that sounds spiritual. Rather, when it starts to come about, encourage it and make the space for it to happen, whether it's in your home or outside the home.

When it comes to spiritual practice, which I will give some brief examples of below, again, it is about creating the space for it to happen and honoring that space. Sometimes it will be creating or setting aside an actual physical space and other times it will be about creating the safe place for it to happen.

Do Not Indoctrinate

A common mistake I have found that is made when it comes to spirituality is the tendency we have — especially as adults — to try and sway people to our position, or worse, dismiss others' perspectives. I would ask one favor of the adults reading this book, if you feel you cannot engage with regard to spirituality without indoctrinating, without trying to sway teens to your way of thinking, hold off engaging until you can. I do not ask this from a place of condescension, I ask this from a place of knowing how difficult it can be. Caring, passionate adults want so badly to share something that works for them or that is part of their lives that it can be hard not to get overzealous.

I'm asking this of parents too. What? You're going to tell me I cannot share my practices or raise my teen/s how I see fit? Of course you can share your practices, and yes, you do have the right to raise your teen/s as you see fit. I would ask that as you do so, try not to cut off every other avenue of spirituality. I have witnessed how doing so caused strained relationships and much turmoil.

As I share these next recommendations with you, it is really about what has worked and what can work. None of these practices should be approached from a place of limitation.

Meditation

Here he goes with the hippy-dippy stuff. Maybe so; however, I would argue that all of us meditate on some level and probably do not realize we are doing it. Dan Millman, in his book "Everyday Enlightenment," talks about the idea of making everything a meditation, like doing laundry, taking out the trash or just sitting. The idea is that you are bringing complete focus and awareness to everything you are doing. When you are doing laundry, you are completely focused on it; the feel, the smell, how your body is moving, etc. Above, I gave the example of riding a motorcycle as a spiritual experience. Part of that is because of what some riders describe and what Dan Millman suggests as everything being a meditation.

I will say here and now that the above idea can be very appealing to teens and in some ways it is easier for them to get into this habit. Teens feel things intensely. They get immersed in their experiences and this is sometimes mistaken by adults, who are trying to get their attention, as a lack of respect or being dismissive. Again, the idea is bringing awareness to every part of your body, to be totally focused on what is happening through all the senses. While I have found teens to be especially good at this, it does take some practice and getting used to.

There are also many other forms of meditation from what the word tends to conjure up; sitting in a lotus position or chanting a mantra to guided practices and systems of meditation. I do not profess deep knowledge of every single form of meditation and cannot say do this one over that. What I can offer is, when I have worked with teens with meditation, both as described above and with a more formal practice led either by myself or another practitioner, we found it opened up avenues for spiritual health.

One thing that meditation does for teens is that it opens up a way to understand their mind and create that space for reflecting on a purpose higher than themselves. I know that was the case of Olivia, a high school senior at the time, who came to me feeling completely frenetic and confused about what she was seeing around her. Olivia came from a family that was not very spiritual; not so much because they didn't want to be, they just hadn't considered it as an important part of their lives. It goes without saying that we worked on more than just meditation. We both found that meditation really helped raise her spiritual health, especially the idea of everything being a meditation.

"Before I started doing this, I would just sort of do what I needed to but didn't always pay full attention. I didn't really know that I could be aware of everything I was doing with, like, almost every part of me. I think this helped me see that there is more than just doing the everyday things; maybe there is something more. I do feel like I care about things more, like really everything, but I'm not stressed about it."

Meditation has opened up a pathway for many teens that I have worked with and it does have the added benefits, as Olivia described, of stress reduction and increasing focus and attention.

Martial Arts/Yoga

As I mentioned in the section on exercise, martial arts and yoga also can have a spiritual dimension to them. Not every form of these two great systems has a spiritual component and not every practitioner delves into the spiritual aspect, but many do.

I would again recommend Tai Chi and Qi Gong as well as yoga. What I suggest that the teens I work with look for in a practitioner is someone who talks about and practices the spiritual aspects. Most studios and schools allow prospective participants to sit in on at least one free class, if not more. That's when you would really get to see what takes place and if it will provide the desired spiritual component. I also suggest finding out what the school or dojo's focus is. Is it about getting students into and winning competitions? Is it a hyped-up excuse for machismo and condoning physical or other forms of dominance over another? This seems to be less common in yoga.

Most schools and dojos are 100% reputable and well meaning; some aren't and the same goes for practitioners. I tend to let teens sniff this out for themselves, as they have a good nose for who's real and who isn't. A quick example is a teen I was working with who was considering a particular martial arts dojo that we both had heard a few positive things about. He was all set to participate in a free class until he came upon the Facebook page of the dojo. As he scrolled through, he found that the owner called himself a warrior and had photos of himself in intentionally intimidating and dominating postures. One included one with the owner posing with his heavily tattooed arms folded in what was supposed to be an intimidating pose.

Mind you, there is nothing wrong with tattoos at all; some of my best friends have multiple tattoos. However, this, along with the postures and the warrior assertion, really turned this particular teen off. There is also nothing wrong with the term 'warrior'; however, it seemed to this teen that all things taken together went against the spirituality of the martial art. To be clear, none of these are an indication of a bad or unscrupulous practitioner or has any inherent issue attached. It was just that for this teen it wasn't right.

I want to be careful about presenting this in a way that seems the only reason to participate in martial arts or yoga is for the spiritual aspect. It's not. In fact, teens can get what they need for their spiritual health from other endeavors and can take martial arts or yoga for the many other health benefits.

Breathing

Isn't breathing just another form or even part of meditation? Yes, in fact, it is said that the simplest form of meditation is paying attention to your breath, and no, in that whether or not it's true that paying attention to your breath is the simplest form of mediation or that breathing is part of meditation. Breathing in and of itself is different.

Focusing on ways of breathing and how you breathe opens up an awareness to spirituality. In a very real sense, in opens up the pathways for spiritual health. There are some very simple breathing exercises one can do and I would also recommend any techniques by Andrew Weil or Deepak Chopra in this area. Many of us are familiar with the idea of taking a deep breath. I recommend doing this as often as possible. There is some dispute over whether to breathe in through your mouth or nose when doing this. I find it doesn't matter so long as deep breaths are taken where the diaphragm expands.

Another interesting idea that Andrew Weil speaks about is an idea taken from Eastern philosophies that exhalation, breathing out, is actually the start of the breath cycle instead of inhalation, breathing in, as we tend to think of it in the West. The idea is that exhalation expels air, which then allows your lungs to fill up; the more air exhaled, the more air and oxygen inhaled.

This does take practice, but it's something that teens have had good success with.

Another simple technique, as mentioned above, is simply noticing one's breath. When I introduce this to teens, I tell them to just notice their breath without trying to control it. This sometimes makes them — or really anyone — try to control it, but once they can bring gentle attention back to noticing their breath, they can get the hang of it. It does help to focus on feeling the breath, either in the mouth or nose. This simple technique brings awareness to the breath, and again, opens up pathways for spiritual health.

When Angelo came to see me, he had been struggling for a while with feelings of despair. He and his mother told me that he did not see the point in anything. He described it as being lost. We had some other work to do besides breathing, but from both his and my own perspective, the breathing is what started to open him up.

We started with having him just notice his breath and then we talked about what it was like. At first, there wasn't much of a noticeable difference. As we continued and used exhalation as the start of the breathing cycle, there began to be some changes. He came in one day, sat down, smiled and asked me how I was doing. You might be thinking, big deal, everybody does that. For Angelo, smiling was uncommon and he had never asked me how I was doing in all of our previous meetings. When I asked him the simple question, "What's up?" he said, "I realized that everything breathes in one way or another, especially people. It's like that's what everyone is trying to do, to breathe. Everyone has to. Maybe everything has to. When I feel like I can't, it messes everything else up; maybe it messes everyone else up too."

There was more than just working with the breath at play here, but I really believe this was the gateway. This above conversation would have never happened without it, nor would the rest of the work we did together.

Remember to breathe deeply, my friends.

Chapter Six

Mental & Emotional Health

Mental and emotional health are intrinsically connected, though they can be thought of separately. In general, mental health is thought of as healthy mental processing, like thinking, reasoning, rational thought, processing information and decision making. Emotional health is generally more about emotions, like angry, sad, happy, joyful, worried, love, compassion, as well as processing and expressing those emotions. For teens, this can be especially challenging, given the barrage of emotions they experience and how quickly they can change.

The connection between thoughts and feelings can be hard to separate. We know that emotions can affect thoughts and thoughts can affect emotions. We know too that thoughts and emotions can manifest physically. For example, teens may think that their friend 'looks depressed' because of the physical changes they have noticed. Though some may disagree, this doesn't mean that you can't have a thought without having an emotion attached to it. In fact, I would say that this happens quite often and in some way is a measure of knowing what is important to you.

With teens, I will ask them to think about certain scenarios or topics to see if there is any emotion attached to it. It helps them gauge importance and is a good idea of what it really means to them. Thinking and feeling are connected, but not to the point where one can never exist without the other.

So what is mental health or good mental health? This is the crux of a lot of my work with teens or anyone of any age for that matter. This, again, is an area that I emphasize with teens, because it's fundamental to support good mental health practices during this time and because I recognize their challenges. One major challenge is the example of mental health that teens see in the media. As the U.S. is currently in the midst of a presidential campaign and election cycle, this dearth of positive examples are readily apparent.

Teens are at that wonderful place of starting to understand and observe the adult world, contemplating what it means to be an adult and what kind of adult they want to be and will be, while still being firmly grounded in their teen years. Teens look to adults for some sort of framework. They observe and sort through the myriad of examples of mental health that adults put out there. This doesn't mean teens shouldn't take responsibility for their actions or that they don't have free will, it just means that they will have to sort through what they take in and see in the media and real life in order to understand it.

The study of mental health is a discipline unto itself. It would take a much more in-depth exploration than there is room for in this chapter to cover all the aspects of mental health. Indeed, one could dedicate their entire life to the study of mental health and luckily many have. Below are some common components of mental health and ones that have been important in my work with teens.

Sometimes referred to as cognition thinking, in terms of mental health, it's more or less the habits we develop or thoughts that become automatic or primary. Thinking is not limited to these habits. They are just, in general, the first thoughts or constructs we have a tendency towards.

Metacognition is sometimes referred to as thinking about thinking or thinking about one's own thinking. For the most part, this is where changes in thinking can arise as knowledge is gained about one's own thinking processes. Sometimes this is also referred to as introspection, which is the ability to reflect on one's thoughts and how those thoughts lead to certain behaviors.

In the teen years, this ability to reflect upon one's own thinking or being introspective is developing and being honed. This is such an exciting time because no longer are teens just going along or simply reflecting the thoughts of the adults around them. Teens are truly starting to form new patterns of thinking; not necessarily rejecting or replacing old ones, but adding to them.

In the recommendations section, I will provide some examples and suggestions on what has worked to foster thinking in the general sense and metacognition. What I will say here is that support is key. Metacognition and forming new thinking patterns can at first be a bit confusing and throw teens off a little. While teens tend to gravitate more towards their friends, having adult support and understanding is important as this type of thinking unfolds.

When you form logical conclusions based on facts and proof, then you are said to be reasoning or using reason. There are types of reasoning like comparative, conditional, deductive and inductive reasoning. There is also a process of reasoning which uses observation, fact, inference, assumption, opinion, argument and critique. The scientific method, in a very real way, depends on inductive reasoning, where you make a generalization or a rule based on observations and inferences and it can be used to make predictions, and deductive reasoning starts out with a general premise and makes specific conclusions.

A quick example of the reasoning process is, you're walking alone down a street and you observe a woman walking a dog. The dog barks and runs towards every person who passes by. The woman holds the dog on the leash so that the dog does not actually make contact with anyone. From this you predict that the dog will bark and run towards you as you pass by. Then you make a decision on what you will do; cross the street, keep walking as you have been, stop, etc. Most likely, you will create an argument to defend your reasoning and reflect on the outcome. Depending on how it turns out, you may stay with or change your behavior.

Some of this process depends on previous experiences and often we will make inferences or reasoning based on past experiences. This is natural but can cause a problem if we do not consider changing our conclusions or behavior in light of new evidence. Using the above example, if you decided to stoop down to pat the dog and the dog suddenly bit you, that is new evidence that you didn't have before. In light of this new evidence, you can decide to change the action you take the next time you encounter a dog exhibiting the same or similar behavior. A logical conclusion would be considering changing your behavior or actually changing your behavior. As in, the last time I got bit when this happened, so this time I will not stoop down to pat the dog. None of this means that every time you encounter a dog acting this way it will play out in the same way.

As teens are gathering experiences, they will likely integrate these experiences into their process of reasoning. This I believe to be a very important area for teens. Teens seek and some would say crave new experiences. This, for the most part, is wonderful. Though, when craving new experiences, if the reasoning process breaks down, it can lead to bad choices or mistakes that can be serious. Adults, unfortunately, do not always model this in the best way, often sticking to old ways of doing things or preconceived notions. This can be confusing for teens but can be worked through with support and understanding.

Rational Thought

When one is thinking rationally, they consider all the relevant variables of a situation and then gather, sort and analyze relevant information to come to a conclusion. This differs a bit from reasoning in that one is usually not approaching the situation with any preconceived rules or generalizations. I would add that rational thought also includes considering multiple perspectives. When considering multiple perspectives, one is able to look at the relevant information presented from all sides and also consider why that might be important. I would also add that rational thought is being able to bring together all relevant information and perspectives to come to a rational conclusion. Action doesn't always follow, but it often does. In short, this means that considering the facts along with multiple perspectives makes up rational thought.

Emotions can affect rational thought. Teens get a bad rap because their emotions sometimes get in the way of rational thinking. While this isn't a revelation by any means, this happens with adults too. The key is to be able to get back on track to understand that emotion can impact rational thought. Some would argue that rational thought is exactly that, thought without emotion, and it is. The tricky part is knowing when emotion is trying to creep in and being able to put it aside. I will go into further detail on emotional health in the next section.

For teens, rational thought is something they can be very good at given the opportunity. I want to note that, as of late, good examples of rational thought are getting harder to find, but they do exist.

Decision Making

In his book "Brainstorm: The Power and Purpose of the Teenage Brain," Dr. Daniel J. Siegel points out that there is an increase in the amount of dopamine released in the teenage brain. In essence, dopamine is a neurotransmitter that fuels our drive for reward. We can imagine how this impacts decision making for teens. Teens are certainly capable of making good decisions and often do. However, we do know that teens can be rather impulsive at times, and as Dr. Siegel explains, this is in part due to the increased release and receptivity of dopamine.

The impulsivity of teens is often a blessing, as they are not overanalyzing a situation and may be more likely to try something new and expand their experiences. On the other hand, this can lead to bad decisions, some of which can have a serious impact on teen health and happiness. Something to consider is that not all decisions have the same importance and what may seem trivial to an adult takes on major importance for a teen. Adults sometimes forget what it was like for them to be a teen and some choose to ignore what they experienced during their teenage years. Because of this, they don't always recognize that for a teen missing a phone call, a text, a Tweet or social event can be a big deal.

Most teens I have worked with don't like hearing this part, but sometimes they do need help making good decisions; other times they don't. The good news is that, in my experience, most teens are pretty good at knowing when they need to seek adult help and guidance. Much to the chagrin of adults, they don't always go to a parent or guardian, as it depends on the type of relationship the teen has with the adult and whether they trust the adult to take them seriously and not pass judgment.

When teens are given the space to think, reason and use rational thought, they often arrive at good decisions. Sometimes, though, the drive for reward, which can lead to impulsiveness, interferes with this process. Such is the beauty of the teen years.

So What Do We Do Now?

How do we support good mental health in teens? For one, it's a good idea to talk with teens and give them space to talk about it if we can be honest about what good mental health is and what the above aspects of mental health look like.

As stated earlier, examples of good mental health are hard to find, at least with respect to pop culture and the media. It seems that teens are bombarded with images and examples of wild exaggerations, false claims, rejection of scientific evidence with nothing more than opinion and faulty reasoning. It's a good idea to talk through these instances with teens when the opportunities arise. It doesn't need to be and shouldn't be forced. Teens will often comment on what they see and hear, so that can be a good time for dialog.

Part of developing these aspects of good mental health is practice. Assuredly, teens know how to think, reason, engage in rational thought and make decisions. Like anything, having the opportunities to practice and engage in these activities allows teens to further develop their mental muscles. The challenge is always how to do this in a way that is natural and builds on what teens can already do.

As we did in the previous chapter, a good place to start is with the questions below. In case you aren't reading this book chapter by chapter, I will provide some suggestions about how to approach answering these questions.

These questions are not about a right or wrong answer. Don't worry about what you think the answers are supposed to be; just answer as honestly as you can. It's about bringing awareness to what is happening and having time for reflection. You may find that just answering these questions provides new insight or a new perspective.

So whether you're a teen or adult reading this book, the questions are here to get you to think about your mental and emotional health habits and what they look like. If you're an adult that isn't a parent to teens but works with teens, answer the questions based on what you have observed from working with teens.

As with all the questions in this book, grab a piece of paper and a pen, get comfortable, sit back, relax and have fun answering the following questions:

- *Question 1:* Based on the above aspects of mental health, how would you describe the teen/s in your life's mental health?
- *Question 2:* Describe the teen/s in your life's intellectual pursuits.
- *Question 3:* How would you describe the teen/s in your life's ability to reason?
- *Question 4:* Would you consider the teen/s in your life to be a rational/rational thinker/s? Why?
- *Question 5:* How would you describe the teen/s in your life's decision-making skills?

As with all the questions in this book, I suggest revisiting these questions from time to time to note any changes and to see your progress. These questions are merely a guide to exploration and I invite you to come up with your own.

I offer the following recommendations based on my work with teens in the field that will offer some insight into the above questions.

Recommendations/Examples

Intellectual Pursuits

Perhaps one of the aspects teens need most for good mental health is intellectual pursuits. I don't mean highbrow activities that are exclusionary or intellectual snobbery. I mean pursuits that primarily involve using one's mind more so than one's body, but this doesn't mean one can't use their body during an intellectual pursuit either. The intellectual pursuits also need to be challenging; not so challenging that the teens cannot engage, but challenging enough so that it stretches their thinking and keeps them interested. Teens that are in school or homeschooled do engage in intellectual pursuits; however, what I am referring to here are more personalized intellectual pursuits, ones that are less prescriptive, time sensitive or overmeasured.

I profoundly believe that teens do not get enough time to do this, nor is it encouraged by our dominant culture. Teens are overscheduled and overprescribed in an attempt to rack up more accomplishments or AP class credits. I know that there is a real void for teens in this area. In fact, I would say that in my work with teens, it's one of the most common areas where teens are lacking.

Gerry came to me after a very difficult eighth grade year. He felt that he was doing a lot but getting nowhere. For all he knew, all the things he did were not really part of anything. His story is typical in that teens are expected to do everything so they can create some sort of portfolio so that they can go to the next step. As Gerry and I worked together, we found that what he was craving was some sort of intellectual challenge that he would come to on his own. We set out to come up with a list of intellectual pursuits, making sure that we agreed upon the caveat that it had to have the right amount of challenge too. What we came up with was Gerry spending his time creating a book of problems to be solved by teens ranging from math problems to moral dilemmas. After about six weeks, we noticed that the way in which Gerry was talking about life in general started to become more positive and he felt that his contribution had meaning.

Of course, there are many other intellectual pursuits like reading, writing, art, music, playing chess, problem solving, inventing and so on. Again, the challenge has to be in the right balance. Take reading, for example, choosing a text that has challenging ideas, not just challenging words, is important. The ideas need to be accessible and not too far outside the reach of the reader.

Make time for, encourage and give the teen space to choose his or her intellectual pursuits.

Experiences

We all have a need for experiences and we learn best through experiences. This is sometimes referred to as experiential learning. In the context of mental health, experiences help teens use reason and rational thought and also helps them to make good decisions. A critical part of this is having the time to be able to reflect upon their experiences.

As teens reflect upon their experiences, they often have to think and reason and use rational thought, especially if they are reflecting on decisions they have made. Not all experiences are necessarily good ones, but real experiences will give teens the chance to practice thinking, reasoning and rationalizing. Since teens naturally seek out new experiences, this is a natural marriage.

Responsibility

In today's culture, most teens are not given much real responsibility. They are overprotected and deemed by most adults to be untrustworthy when it comes to making good decisions. We ask youth to spend the first 18 to 19 years of their life having little responsibility and less say, with the most important decisions being made for them by adults. Then suddenly after 18 or 19 years of this, we turn them loose and expect them to know how to make good decisions. This doesn't work very well and causes these 18- to 19-year-olds unnecessary stress.

Teens know when they aren't given any real responsibility or aren't allowed to make important decisions. In turn, this causes resentment and a sense of helplessness. When I talk with adults about this, a common question I get is whether I think teens should be able to make all the decisions related to them. This depends on the age of the teen and on how often they have made important decisions in the past.

It would be unfair and unwise to go from the teen making no important decisions to making all of them. The earlier the teen or preteen is allowed to make decisions, the better their decision-making ability becomes. It is better to have them make decisions and possible mistakes while they have the support and safety net of caring adults. Often, adults mistakenly try to insulate teens from responsibility or the possibility of making a bad decision. When teens don't have the practice, they will likely not make the best of decisions once they are out on their own. In terms of developing good mental health, giving teens responsibility will help them become more responsible for their behavior and learn to make better decisions.

When Jenna came to me, she expressed frustration with what she felt was a lack of trust and 'babying' from her parents. "I know they care about me and want to protect me, but they treat me like a baby. I can't make any decisions on my own — well, not any big ones anyway. They want me to start thinking about colleges, but now I don't know if I will make the right decision."

Jenna also felt that her parents would make the decision for her if she didn't choose a college fast enough. This is the kind of decision-making paralysis that is common in today's teens, but it does not have to be. I worked with Jenna's parents to give her more responsibility; however, it never really got to the point where she was making real, important decisions for herself. In the end, in part with my help, she did choose a college, but did so, I felt, under needless pressure because she had waited so long to do so.

Responsibility and decision making also helps teens get to know themselves well, to know what they really want or at least what that is at the time. I believe Jenna would've had an easier time with her decision had she been given more responsibility, as she would have known herself better and what she really wanted to pursue.

Spend Time In Nature

As I will expand more on the benefits of spending time in nature in another chapter, I will keep this section brief.

In short, one of the best things teens can do to support their mental health and overall health and happiness is to spend time in nature. Some may think this is only realistic for those who live in the suburbs or rural areas. Most urban areas have some sort of park or green space, and if you can't find one, you can create one. Teens need this in a big way.

One of my main gripes with the way most school days are structured is that they allow for little to no time outdoors in nature. I am not talking about going outside in PE class, though that is a positive thing. I mean, getting a chance to spend time in a natural area. The research is clear on the need for humans of any age to spend time in nature. In my work with teens, it is clear how much they need and want this. They don't always know they want it until they get the chance to experience it. I will expand upon this idea further in another chapter.

Emotional Health

The teen years are usually marked by a flood of intense and varying emotions. This is completely normal, though perhaps frustrating to teens and adults. Many caricatures and not so flattering representations of the 'moody teen' abide in our culture. Though these are often exaggerated, they do bring to light the nature of teen emotions.

Teens have highs and lows in their emotions and these seem to change rapidly with little reason. Shifting hormones are certainly part of the mix and in reality that is part of being a teenager. It can be difficult for teenagers to regulate or rationally deal with the intense emotions they feel, especially when they are new experiences. Younger children experience emotions as well; however, theirs are not as intense or fluctuating. This is in no way an attempt to downplay the very real emotions younger children feel or suggest that they should be taken less seriously.

If we pause to think about the amount of variation in the emotions teens feel on a daily basis, they actually do pretty well working with them. A common phrase I hear is 'helping teens manage their emotions'. And while there is genuine sentiment in this, it is a bit limiting. I have watched many adults approach teen emotions from this standpoint and gloss over the need for teens to actually feel their emotions. If emotions are always suppressed, how can we expect them to work with them? Again, I will say that many of the examples teens see in media and pop culture are detrimental to teen emotional health and their overall health and happiness

I describe below some aspects of emotional health that have been critical in my work with teens.

Understanding Ups & Downs

When teens understand that the ups and downs in their emotions are natural, it is easier for them to process their emotions. Their emotions do change rapidly; however, this doesn't mean that they won't get caught up in their emotional state.

Teens are not always aware of how often their emotions fluctuate, so it is helpful when we can use examples or simply ask about the range of emotions they feel on a given day. It also helps for teens to know that hormones play a role in the ups and downs they feel. When they are given a bit more knowledge about themselves, especially in this area, it is empowering. I know that when teens can make peace with the ups and downs and know this is a natural part of being a teen, they feel more in control.

An important point to make here is that while it is normal for teens to experience ups and downs or be 'moody', there are times of stability. So if a teen's emotions seem to always have severe highs and lows and/or are severely disproportional to situations, then it may be a sign of something more serious. Adults can be helpful in this area if they, themselves, embrace the ups and downs of teen emotions and try not to take them personally.

We all receive a plethora of messages that tell us to suppress our emotions or just put them on the side and do your job, go to school, etc. Some of that is actually okay. Sometimes it does help to not let our emotions overrun us to the point where it stops us from participating in our daily lives. On the other hand, when this is the dominant message teens receive, that their emotions are something to be shunned or that if they actually feel their emotions, they are somehow defective, it creates teens that shy away from feeling their emotions, trying to cover up or put on a brave face.

This is especially true for teenage boys, who are on their way to manhood in a society that tells men showing or feeling or any kind of emotion means they are less of a man. Add in the message that men need to be emotionally available in romantic relationships and it's no wonder teens are sometimes confused about what to do with their emotions.

Encouraging teens to feel their emotions helps them understand what they're feeling and why. This doesn't mean wallowing in their emotions or using emotions as an excuse for negative behaviors is okay. The reality is that when teens feel their emotions, it can be intense, but trying to repress those emotions very likely leads to them manifesting in other ways that aren't so positive.

The time teens take to feel their emotions is important. If adults can provide this time and be understanding of this need, it will go a long way in teens getting in touch with their emotions.

Part of emotional health is also being able to process emotions in healthy ways. This may sound a little stale or clinical to say 'processing emotions'. Primarily, this means working towards understanding your emotions, where they are coming from and what, if anything, you need to do with them.

Of course, one of the first steps is being able to feel emotions. Once we feel the emotion, we try to identify what that emotion is and the cause of that emotion. This can be more challenging than it seems and is unquestionably challenging for teens. For instance, for some teens when they are feeling angry, they think it's just that, anger. When they look a little deeper, they understand the reason for their anger, which could be betrayal, hurt, shame and a host of other emotions that may be at the root of their anger.

Once we have identified the emotion and the reason for that emotion, we decide what action to take, if any. We don't always need to take action, as sometimes the emotion will pass without having to take a specific action. As I've worked with teens on this, we would, at times, come to the point where the energy of the emotion needed to go somewhere. Much of that time we spent looking at ways to shift the focus and look at all angles and perspectives behind that emotion. This is not easy, but it is definitely possible.

When teens process emotions in the fashion outlined above or in other ways, they are learning and experiencing important coping skills. Adults can model this process, as it is helpful for teens to see adults do this. I would say though, the most important part is giving teens the space to process their emotions. It's what they need the most. Well-meaning adults sometimes forget this important aspect and try moving things along too quickly. Teens, like any age group, also, at times, need space to get to a place where they can do the work of processing their emotions.

So What Do We Do Now?

Knowing and accepting the fact that teens have intense and varying emotions helps teens and adults keep perspective. Teens and adults can embrace teenage emotions rather than avoid them. To be clear, embracing emotions is not a green light to use emotions as a shield or excuse for poor behavior. It is a way forward, a way for teens to feel, express, understand and process their emotions.

There's no question that working through teen emotions will be difficult at times for both adults and teens. That being said, the emotions must be worked with in a way that promotes good emotional health. A key point to remember is that emotions are not always predictable and the process of dealing with them is imperfect. Sometimes things will go awry. When this happens, just acknowledge that they have and get back on track. For any adults reading this book, I can tell you that teens appreciate your understanding and your ability to not take their emotions personally. They truly crave understanding and a safe space to be present with their emotions.

I remember chatting with Kate, a then 15-year-old, and after about five minutes asked how she was doing. She immediately broke into tears, and despite my best efforts, our time ended with her leaving in sobs. Our next few interactions were awkward, as she was distant and even purposefully mean. Admittedly, I was confused but didn't try to push the issue or force a conversation. I just gave her the space she needed. Eventually, we were able to talk about what happened. This, in some ways, is a good illustration of teens' fluctuating emotions.

Kate was very appreciative of my understanding and patience and my respect of her need for space. "Adults don't get it. We (teens) get confused or we can be in a bad mood, but it isn't really about them. You know, I have adults think I'm a bad person because I didn't feel like talking to them, but they didn't notice I didn't feel like talking to anybody. Now when I try to talk to them or be nice to them, they treat me different. Thank you for not doing that."

We need to take the rollercoaster of teen emotions seriously and also be flexible enough to extend understanding and patience to teens as they go along for the ride.

As we have been doing throughout this book, we have used some questions to get the conversation started. In case you aren't reading this book chapter by chapter, I have been providing some suggestions about how to approach answering these questions.

Of course, you do not have to use any of them. These questions are not about a right or wrong answer. Don't worry about what you think the answers are supposed to be; just answer as honestly as you can. It's about bringing awareness to what is happening and having time for reflection. You may find that just answering these questions provides new insight or a new perspective.

So whether you're a teen or adult reading this book, the questions are here to get you to think about your or the teen/s in your life's emotional health and what it looks like. If you're an adult that isn't a parent to teens but works with teens, answer the questions based on what you have observed from working with teens.

As with all the questions in this book, grab a piece of paper and a pen, get comfortable, sit back, relax and have fun answering the following questions.

- *Question 1:* How would you describe the teen/s in your life's emotional health?
- *Question 2:* Given the discussion in this chapter on emotional health, is there anything about the teen/s in your life's emotions that seems outside the range of what was discussed?
- *Question 3:* How do you discuss emotional health with the teen/s in your life?
- *Question 4:* What is/are the teen/s in your life's comfort level with their emotions?
- *Question 5:* How does/do the teen/s in your life process their emotions?

As with all the questions in this book, I suggest revisiting these questions from time to time to note any changes and to see your progress. These questions are a guide to exploration and I invite you to come up with your own.

I offer the following recommendations for emotional health based on my work with teens in the field that will offer some insight into the above questions.

Recommendations/Examples

Expression

Teens need to express their emotions. Again, this doesn't mean they can and should do it in a negative way. Teens are often brimming with emotions just waiting to be expressed. Sometimes just the act of expressing emotions provides insight and a feeling of relief.

There are many ways to express emotion and it doesn't have to be done through talking. Writing, creating a piece of art or performing an action are some great ways to express emotion. Given the chance, teens are often creative in finding ways to express their emotions. It is a need that gets overlooked at times because there are so many demands on teenagers. Adults don't always realize that teens aren't getting the chance to express their emotions.

Tyler, a college freshman, explained it to me in this way, "I know that I need to express my emotions like we talked about. I think I need more time to do that. Either I am not making the time or my schedule doesn't allow me to do that. I know that I was in high school, and even though I am officially an adult, adults didn't always understand that I needed a chance or maybe time and space to express my emotions. I have ways that I do that when I get the chance to,"

Practice

When I talk about practicing good strategies for emotional health, I, at times, get raised eyebrows. I do mean taking opportunities to practice processing and working with emotions. I don't mean setting a schedule to do so or trying to force it on teens. I recommend starting with less intense situations when emotions are not quite so high. From there, the teen can practice feeling, identifying and processing their emotions.

The important point here is to make this about learning about themselves and how they can work with their emotions.

De-stressing

Stress can wreak havoc on emotional health. Stress can be a result of unexpressed or unresolved emotions. It can also be from the demands of the outside world. Teens are not immune to stress, as some seem to feel. I dare to say that teens can and do feel stress at least as deeply as adults. Sure, I have heard 'what do teens have to be stressed about' from adults who have forgotten what it was like for them or don't want to concede that being a teen today comes with more pressure and scrutiny.

I worked with a group of teens in a boarding facility that was highly demanding; designed that way on purpose to limit downtime and the temptation to fall back into destructive habits during that downtime. The stress levels would build and the teens would need a way to de-stress. As we were sitting together in a group one day, we started to talk about the stress they were feeling. We talked about how stress can build if we don't manage it. They started to tell me about how they could feel the stress around them and how they felt it became a barrier to good emotional health.

Jose said, "They (the adults at the school) think we are machines. Every part of our day is scheduled. I know why, Bro. I know why, but it makes me stress out. We don't get time to get our stress out. We do get to play sports or run around, but it's not enough. It makes it harder to make good decisions or, you know, be patient when I'm stressed."

Teens need ways to deal with the stress in their lives. Already in this book we have touched on ways to manage stress. Some of those include good nutrition, exercise and movement and paying attention to spiritual and mental health. Other recommendations are walking, talking with friends, seeing a funny movie, listening to music, cooking, spending time with pets and engaging in physical labor.

Journaling

One of my all-time favorite recommendations is journaling. This does not have to be a written journal. It can be audio or video recordings or can be accomplished by using speech-recognition software. Journaling in any of these forms or in another form is one of the best ways to work through emotions. It works nicely for teens, as they learn about how they process emotions and what ways work best for them to express and embrace their emotions. It's also a great way to practice processing emotions. A journal is not meant to be just one more thing a teen has to do, but a private place for them to reflect on their emotional health. Teens can share their journal with adults if the choose. Adults should respect a teen's need for privacy and should not violate that unless they must for the safety of the teen.

There isn't a particular format that works best. It just has to be a place where teens can truly reflect and work through their emotions. The journal is best used and viewed as a positive addition to teens' lives. As it can take various forms, it generally appeals to teens of any gender. I have had really good success with journaling. In fact, it is one of the first things I recommend when I work with teens in most capacities.

Ian, a high school senior, came to enjoy his journaling time. His preferred method was making short video recordings on his smartphone. I suggested that he offload the videos and store them somewhere that only he had access to. He started to cherish journaling, as it gave him time to reflect and just talk freely about his emotions. From time to time, I would give him prompts to talk about or just ask him how it was going. He always seemed eager to share his stories. He felt that journaling gave him a healthy way to process his emotions in a way that nothing else had.

"When you first brought up journaling, I wasn't happy. I thought that meant I was going to have to write. I don't have anything bad against writing; it's just that I write a lot in school. I was glad that I could make recordings on my phone. Now I see that I can express myself in the way that I want to and it really helps. Usually, by the end of journaling, I feel better and sometimes I feel like I understand myself better."

Journaling can be a great tool to support good emotional health in teens and overall health and happiness.

Chapter Seven

Relationships

All humans want to come into relationship with each other in some fashion. So much of our culture is focused on relationships in one form or another. This represents the need we all have to forge some type of relationship with people.

Some bring up the idea of being an introvert as a counter to this, but being an introvert is not the absence of relationships; in fact, introverts are more likely to have deep, connected relationships. Most of us do have a need to go into ourselves or have alone time, yet when we emerge from that space, we want to reconnect or at least know that we can connect with others. I, myself, can probably be classified as an extroverted introvert. I value all of my relationships; many I have had for most of my life. I do enjoy the company of others and am generally comfortable in most social situations; however, I do have the need to get introverted or have time to recharge.

During the teen years, the pull to be with their peer group or friends is powerful. Many of the relationships formed during this time period are intense and often last well into adulthood. Relationships can be challenging, and for teens they are even more challenging, in that along with all the other changes, the nature of their relationships change with adults, peers, children, society and even themselves. It's also exciting and rewarding for the exact same reasons.

I have heard that there are many reasons why people of all ages want to be in relationships, from filling internal emptiness, to a feeling of being taken care of. Relationships at some level may indeed do this, but I believe from my experience that relationships are mostly about sharing and receiving love. Some relationships do help us validate ourselves, while others can tear us down. Teen relationships can be quite intense, especially from an emotional standpoint. In short, teens do care about their relationships, especially the ones that are important to them.

I know that sometimes adults, especially parents, think that the teen/s in their lives don't care about their relationship with them. It's not hard to think that when teens seem so much more interested in their friends and peer group. This is a natural part of being a teen. There are times when relationships between parents and teens get strained. In part, this is a result of how much they care about the relationship with their parents and other adults in their lives. Not to put any added pressure on parents and adults, but teens do care what you think and they care what you think about them.

Just like adults, teens have different types of relationships. They have relationships that are more or less casual, as in people they may interact with and be friendly with but wouldn't be classified as friends, then there are the relationships they have with their friends, siblings, family members and romantic interests.

For most teens there is little time spent on learning about relationships and how to have healthy ones. I have spent a lot of time over the years talking with teens about what it means to have healthy relationships. Below are the major themes from those conversations and also my own observations.

Respect

This seems like a no-brainer; of course we should respect each other. We should respect each other and often do not. For teens this may be even more important than it is for adults to feel respected. This is an area that teens are sensitive to and they can usually sniff out those who do not respect them or are only pretending to respect them.

In order to fully respect someone, you have to view them as having an equal right to be respected. When it comes to teen/adult relationships, I find adults sometimes have a harder time with this than teens. Some adults just don't think teens are entitled to the same respect that they are. They might use an adults-up-here and teens-down-there analogy. That doesn't work.

Before you toss this book in the fire, I want to be clear about what I mean. Sometimes adults need to make decisions about teens and for teens that may be difficult and unpopular. Sometimes — and I would recommend as often as possible — teens should be part of the decision-making process. I go into greater detail on this topic in Chapter Nine. Yes, adults are, at times, put in positions of greater responsibility and their courses of action may have higher stakes attached to them. The truth is, teens are not always going to know, for a variety of reasons, all that goes into decisions adults make.

I am also not suggesting that teens have the run of a household, school or organization without any adult input or guidance. What I am saying is that teens have a right to the same respect that adults do. This means taking them seriously, respecting their right to their opinion — though not necessarily agreeing with it if you really don't, their right not to respect your opinion, their right to ask questions and get real, serious answers that do not play down to them or insult their intellect. This also means that teens need to respect adults in all the same ways mentioned above. The good news is that the vast majority of teens respect adults that respect them.

Liz, a 16-year-old, had this to say, "It's kinda easy. I always respect adults. Sometimes they don't respect me because I'm a teenager and think that I don't know anything. It's hard to respect someone that doesn't respect you and treats you like you're stupid. It's easier when you respect each other."

Teens respecting teens is just as important. Teens are trying things out, trying on new identities and ideas. As teens go through this process, if they can respect each other, give each other a little space, all the while knowing that respecting someone doesn't mean you have to agree with them and at the same time knowing that because you disagree with someone doesn't mean you can disrespect them, they are better off.

Empathy/Compassion

Being able to identify with or take the emotional position of another is known as empathy. This is not feeling sorry for someone; rather, it is understanding or at least doing your best to understand where they are coming from.

Any person appreciates when someone is empathetic and does their best to truly understand their position. I can tell you that teens especially appreciate this from adults. I will be honest and say that it often comes as a surprise to them when they get it from adults. Not because adults don't want to be empathetic, I believe it's because for some adults it's hard to remember what it was like for them to be a teen or to truly understand where the teen is coming from. All I can say is try. Teens will notice and appreciate it.

Teens have an easier time empathizing with their peers since they are likely sharing many of the same experiences. This isn't always the case and it is certainly noticeable when it's absent. Teens can be very concrete or black

113

and white. They're not always able to get outside of themselves to be empathetic and this is where adult guidance can be helpful.

Compassion is closely related to empathy, as it involves understanding how someone feels and taking some kind of action or showing a kindness (as an example, you might offer encouragement to someone who has just suffered a loss or grave disappointment). Teens do have an amazing capacity for compassion, but again, it's not always the case, especially in instances where they are lacking empathy. They need practice with both empathy and compassion and need real opportunities to feel and express it.

Honesty

I can hear the guffaws and can imagine the eye-rolling, as if this is a given. It should be, but as we know, it isn't always. Adults fall into the trap of thinking they need to keep things from teens to protect them. There are a few occasions where that would be warranted. Teens respect and appreciate honesty even more so when it's delivered with empathy and compassion. It's true that teens don't always trust adults and this happens a lot when they feel adults in authority don't tell them the truth. I have always found that teens have a good honesty radar.

I hear a lot from adults that they feel teenagers aren't honest. Like any other group of people, you will get some teens that value honesty more than others. Teens witness so many examples of adult dishonesty that it's hard to expect them not to adopt it in some way, particularly when they notice how adults use it to their benefit. However, healthy relationships are based on honesty and so it is important to be as honest as we can without being unnecessarily cruel. It's also just as important to listen to the honesty of teens

114

without being judgmental or automatically turning it into something punitive. I believe that the more this happens, the more likely it will be that teens will be honest with adults and even their peers. If they fear being judged, misunderstood or otherwise made to feel inadequate or that they will suffer retribution, they will either figure out ways to avoid these interactions or not tell the whole truth.

I have been asked by adults what they should do if they can't tell teens the whole truth for reasons of confidentiality or discretion. The answer there is to simply tell them that. It's the same with teens and their peers. They may not always like that answer, but they will respect it. This also leads to building trust. Teens like to know that they can trust people to keep what they share in confidence. Of course, there are exceptions when what is shared may be harmful to themselves or someone else. If that's the case, let the teen know that.

Listening

We all have a fundamental need to be heard. In fact, we crave this so much that people actually pay others to listen to them. Indeed, much of my work requires listening closely and giving my full attention. It's not always about trying to 'fix the problem', it's listening without judgment. You can always ask a teen if they want help or if they just want to talk. I have had many teens say to me, 'I don't want you to do anything. I just want you to listen.'

Most people know when they are really being listened to and teens are no different. Listening does require full attention. It can be difficult sometimes to just listen if that's all they want, knowing that if you just said this one thing, it might save them a lot of angst. Of course, if teens say they want your help, then by all means give it. There are times when you can ask the teen if you can give them a suggestion.

Another technique is something called paraphrasing or asking for clarity. Paraphrasing is when you are repeating back a shortened version of what is being said, highlighting the main points and checking for understanding. The person, in this case the teen, has a chance to either add or make corrections. You can say something like, 'I want to make sure I understand you're saying that; is that right? Is there more?' At this stage, you have to resist the urge to offer suggestions, unless asked for. In this way you are really listening and understanding what is being said. This also works well for teen-to-teen interactions. It's powerful when adults model this for teens. I know that parents find this to be very helpful and have been surprised by the results.

It's amazing when people feel truly listened to how that can transform a relationship. Listening is an essential component of a healthy relationship, so practice and engage in it as much as you can.

Romantic Relationships

To the chagrin of many adults, the teen years seem to be heavily focused on romantic relationships. Since this does take on greater importance during the teen years, I wanted to briefly discuss them here.

The same underpinnings of healthy relationships discussed above apply to romantic relationships; perhaps even more so. In today's world, everything seems to be about romantic relationships; how everyone should want one and in the exact way the media and our dominant and even fringe culture says we should. If you should buck against these notions, this culture tries to convince you that you're a loser or in some way deficient.

Teens are very susceptible to these suggestions and portrayals, which, at best, are confusing and, at worst, destructive. We don't have enough room in this chapter to name the many examples of popular films and TV that suggest to women and teen girls that they are nothing without a man and to men and teen boys that they are nothing more than how many sexual conquests they can rack up.

There is room to say that this is a problem. Imagine, if you can, a recent TV show, movie or social media page or Internet advertisement that in some way did not center around or reference romantic relationships. Adults can be invaluable here. They can provide guidance and offer space for honest discussion to take place. It's okay for adults to discuss with teens the realities of being in a romantic relationship, although this is not always a comfortable discussion depending on the relationship.

Where things can get even trickier is when these relationships take a turn towards being physically intimate. I am sure we are all familiar with the phrase 'raging teenage hormones' and exaggerated depictions of lustful, promiscuous teens that are nothing more than a collection of cells on hypersexual overdrive. The truth is that, yes, teens are flooded with hormones that bring about sexual desire and that this isn't their only interest or passion. Adults and teens need to understand the difference between how they are depicted and expected to act and the reality of it.

In our culture, almost everything is oversexualized and views and expectations of intimacy distorted and are in no way reflective of reality. Unless one were to totally unplug and avoid any print material with suggestive illustrations or text filled with sexual innuendo, it would be difficult to not be inundated with this oversexualization. With our technological world, we have much at our fingertips. Like the rest of us, teens have around-the-clock access to pretty much anything they are searching for. Even when innocently searching for real information on relationships and sexuality, teens can be bombarded with egregious distortions and purposely-exaggerated imagery.

My time spent with teens leads me to believe that this is another area where adults are needed. These discussions can be awkward, but they are necessary. Honest, real compassionate discussions are critical. Adults can be honest with teens and say it does make them a little uncomfortable, while letting them know they are still committed to being there and being supportive.

I always suggest that unless as an adult you're a licensed professional that needs to discuss this with teens or have parental or legal guardian permission, this is best left to the parents or legal guardian.

So What Do We Do Now?

People and teens, in particular, want and need healthy relationships. Relationships that are built with teens and among teens are paramount to teen health and happiness. Positive relationships have an overall positive impact on teens. The reverse is also true and so the question is, how do adults know when to offer guidance or to intervene?

When there is any confirmed or even suspected form of abuse, whether physical, sexual, verbal or neglect, then it's incumbent on adults or teens to intervene. It's more challenging when the negative impact of a relationship isn't so clear-cut or readily apparent.

Adults have a natural inclination to want to ride in on a white horse and protect teens. I know parents who struggle with wanting to intervene and not wanting to overreach, so much so that they alienate their teenager or fail to allow them to learn from experience. This is where having a healthy relationship with the teen/s in your life will manifest in positive ways. Being able to have an open, respectful, compassionate, empathetic, honest dialog with teens without judgment will keep adults in the loop. This will help with knowing when to give gentle guidance and when to take a firmer stance.

Healthy relationships are an important part of teen health and happiness, and ultimately, they are about self-awareness and the willingness to do the work to have healthy relationships. Teens benefit much from investing energy into having healthy relationships. In all my work with teens and adults, I have had many conversations and have done a lot of work around healthy relationships. The recommendations that follow are the highlights of the result of this work.

First, as we have been doing throughout this book, we will use questions to help with reflection. In case you aren't reading this book chapter by chapter, I have been providing some suggestions about how to approach answering these questions.

Of course, you do not have to use any of them. These questions are not about a right or wrong answer. Don't worry about what you think the answers are supposed to be; just answer as honestly as you can. It's about bringing awareness to what is happening and having time for reflection. You may find that just answering these questions provides new insight or a new perspective.

So whether you're a teen or adult reading this book, the questions are here to get you to think about healthy relationships for teens and adults. If you're an adult that isn't a parent to teens but works with teens, answer the questions based on what you have observed from working with teens.

As with all the questions in this book, grab a piece of paper and a pen, get comfortable, sit back, relax and have fun answering the following questions:

- *Question 1:* How would you describe the relationship between you and the teen/s in your life?
- *Question 2:* What importance do you place on forging healthy relationships with teens? How does this show up?
- *Question 3:* How comfortable are the teens in your life coming to you to talk? How comfortable are you talking with them?
- *Question 4:* How would you describe the communication between you and the teen/s in your life?
- *Question 5:* What are the obstacles to having a healthy relationship with the teen/s in your life?

As with all the questions in this book, I suggest revisiting these questions from time to time to note any changes and to see your progress. These questions are a guide to exploration and I invite you to come up with your own.

I offer the following recommendations for relationships based on my work with teens in the field that will offer some insight into the above questions.

Prioritize/Make Time

Make time to nourish healthy relationships. Make them a priority. This may be sound counterintuitive since the teen years are when teens pull away from adults and focus on the relationships they form with their peer groups. Still, make relationships a priority and don't get discouraged or take it personally if teens don't seem to be making their relationship with you a priority. They will take their cues from you and they will notice and appreciate that your relationship with them is important enough to you that you will set aside time.

In general, teens do make time for relationships and they are a priority for them. When they see how you make time for relationships and the way that you do it, they will borrow from the model you show them. Remember, you don't have to be perfect; you just have to make time for and make relationships with them important.

An instance comes to mind when Conner, a 13-year-old, came to see me. I was sitting at my desk doing some work. When I saw him come in, I immediately got up and sat down at the table with him. I didn't think much of it until the next day when his mother called me. She mentioned how impressed Conner was that I got up from my desk and sat with him. "Conner was so impressed that you got up from your desk and sat down at the table with him to talk. It really is the little things." I offer this here to illustrate that you don't have to make grand gestures to show that a relationship's a priority to you.

Spend time with teens. Get to know their interests and ideas. Take them seriously. Smile. Get personal. Give them real responsibility. Provide space for meaningful discussions. Genuinely care. And have fun. This may all seem like it is aimed at adults who work with teens and not parents, but it works for parents too. Know that what you show is important will become important. However, just making time for and making relationships a priority will not necessarily lead to healthy relationships.

Be Supportive

The teen years are such a wonderful time for many reasons, one of them being the desire to forge meaningful relationships with their peers and, believe it or not, adults too. Parents already have a meaningful (and a good argument can be made for this) and perhaps the most meaningful relationship with teens. The best way that I can put it is that, yes, it is perhaps the most meaningful relationship, but it doesn't always mean it's a healthy relationship.

When I work with teens and parents, a common theme I hear from teens is that they don't feel supported by their parents. I hear many adults say that teens have it too easy and are coddled by their parents to the point where they expect everything to be handed to them and lack resiliency. Many adults adopt the position that teens have too much support. There's a difference between support and doing everything for or constantly intervening on a teen's behalf. Sometimes support means that you let the teen make a mistake and you're there afterwards to help them work through it.

In the chapter on emotional health, we discussed the intense and sensitive nature of teen emotions. Since relationships do have emotions attached to them, relationships for teens take on a special significance, as they can also be a source of disappointment, anxiety and hurt. This is when support becomes most important. I always say to adults and teens that adults need support from teens as well. Adults are people after all and adults need support too. When teens feel supported, they, in turn, will be more likely to support adults. In the end, teens want to feel like adults are in their corner and that doesn't always mean pandering or agreeing, but really being supportive.

Timmy, a tenth grader, told me, "It's a big help when you know that you have adults that support you. I don't always want help from an adult because I want to be able to figure things out on my own, but I like knowing that I have their support."

Balance

When relationships completely consume us, they are not healthy. Didn't you say above that we need to make relationships a priority? I sure did and we need to. What we do not need to do is have relationships consume us. With that said, there are times, as in a crisis or an illness, where it's okay for relationships to consume us for a short while.

Parents assuredly want to provide their teens with everything that they need and make decisions in order to do that. Of course for parents, their kids — teens in this case — are their number-one priority. It is also true that parents need to ensure that they are attending to themselves. Adults that work with teens that aren't their own need to understand how to balance relationships with teens. I have watched well-meaning adults overstep their bounds and wind up burning themselves out because they became overinvested in the relationships they have with teens and didn't know when or even how to separate them.

Anyone who knows me or knows my work may find what I just said surprising. I am an advocate for adults caring very much for the teens in their life. I have dedicated a good portion of my life to doing this. However, like in any relationship, if you get so out of balance to the point where you're not investing in yourself, you'll become ineffective and disappointed.

Most adults that set out to work with teens want to have a positive impact or even change the lives of the teens they work with. This is where things can get easily out of balance. Remember, it's not you who's changing their lives. You may show them the path, clear space for them or extend a hand, but fundamentally, it is the teen that decides whether to take that hand, walk the path or come into the spaces.

Please care about the teens in your life; care about them a lot. Go to bat for them. Walk through the fire with them. Let them fail, succeed, know your limits, and have healthy boundaries and take care of yourself so you can take care of them. This provides a model for teens in their own relationships.

Be Yourself/Let Teens Be Themselves

It is so enriching for teens to be around adults who can be themselves. I get the question, what if that person is a jerk? Should they be themselves? We are going to assume that who you are is not a jerk. Being yourself really is about sharing who you are; your experiences, the things you like and are passionate about. You can share your values with teens so long as you're not trying to convince them that they should share them and respect that they have their own. When teens see that you're being yourself and that you honor

124

who they are, it provides a powerful model. Not only is this a model, it's a real clearing of space for relationships to be authentic.

The teen years are filled with experimentation and sometimes that experimentation isn't always going to be positive. They are trying out who they are and who they are may change. Teens do need to be allowed to be themselves and this is just as important with their peer groups as it is with adults. How great is it when we can be ourselves without the worry of being judged, ridiculed or diminished? If all of the pieces of healthy relationships examined in this chapter are in place, people being themselves would seem like a natural fit.

Chapter Eight

Purpose & Passion

Purpose

In the previous chapter on relationships, we explored the need for healthy relationships. Just as important and related is the real need humans have for purpose. Purpose, or the reason for doing something, is what drives or motivates us. Purpose can also be looked at as something you're aspiring to. Teens have a need for purpose just as adults do. When purpose gets discussed, it can be taken to mean pursuing one's life's purpose or even what their day-to-day purpose is. What I've learned from teens is that purpose or the 'why' can change for them quickly. This is part of their experimentation and exploration.

What is more, teens can, at times, lose purpose or don't always feel that they have purpose. This happens for a few reasons. One is, though we live in a world that is truly globally connected, teens sometimes feel disconnected with the world and with people. Two, teens are not part of conversations about them or for them; they are told explicitly and implicitly they don't have a voice — at least not yet. Three, they are marginalized in society by overexaggerated representations and are regularly not taken seriously.

This is not to say that teens never feel that they have purpose, they do, and the difference is noticeable when they do and when they don't. Luckily, this shifts rapidly, so if teens are feeling like they don't have purpose, it doesn't last, as teens are constantly searching for purpose or meaning. When

126

teens have purpose, motivation or aspirations, they are inspired and often move quickly. As adults, we have to work with that energy and support teens as they move with purpose. In the end, we want teens to feel their own meaning and purpose. They can and do find it.

They do seek adults for this from time to time. Teens, in their search for purpose, may not always go in the direction adults think is best. I assure you, this is natural and it comes down to accepting that searching for and having purpose is as unique as each individual is unique. Stay the course and teens will look to you even if it isn't readily apparent to you.

There is much research that indicates that teens who have purpose — or as is the case for many teens searching for purpose — experience an overall higher degree of happiness. According to teens, the following aspects characterize purpose.

Personal Meaning

A group of teens explained personal meaning to me in this way: 'It's when you know that something is important to you and maybe other people don't think it's important, but you do.' I have been witness to how personalized meaning can be. When it comes to purpose, it's not only in that what is meaningful differs from person to person, it's also that why it's meaningful differs as well. The reason or reasons why any experience or pursuit is personally meaningful are as varied as there are individuals.

As I talked with the group further about how part of purpose has personal meaning, a few more insights came to light. "When I have purpose or a purpose, I guess it feels like this is what I am supposed to do. I want to do it too. It's just — I don't know, it feels like I have to do it. If I didn't, it wouldn't be right." We expanded on this a little more and what was telling is that most of the conversation centered around what personal meaning of purpose felt like.

It would be safe to say then, for the teens I have worked with, purpose is connected with feeling. Another way to express it is, there's a feeling one gets when they have purpose and this is part of where personal meaning comes from. "I think it comes from inside. It's hard to explain, but it feels like I know I really want to be doing that thing. It feels like being happy but serious at the same time."

Connection

Connection, in this sense, is connecting to your purpose in a way that is motivating. Teens say that connecting in this respect is akin to connecting with something bigger than yourself; as such, one's purpose is beyond just them and their immediate surroundings (though teens did express that they felt that's where the most immediate impact may occur).

The idea of purpose being bigger than you or perhaps beyond easy comprehension is a challenging one. When I speak with other adults about this, there is, at times, some pushback; either dismissing it as hokum or stating that there is no way to know when this is happening. I believe that many of us have had the feeling of being connected with something bigger than ourselves and that what we are doing matters to more than just us. In any case, teens have reported this to me and I take these ideas seriously.

When a teen is connected to their purpose, to something bigger than themselves, it is noticeable. The motivation and the commitment comes from inside or is intrinsic. With intrinsic motivation, the teen is not concerned about external rewards or accolades. Their motivation is driven by a sense of internal reward, just doing what they are doing is reward in itself. Spending a lot of time with teens, I have noticed that one of the ways in which this shows up is when teens are not affected by adult feedback. This is not coming from a place of disrespect. It's more so from a place of fulfillment without having to hear from others.

Connection also shows in body language — in the way teens carry themselves, the speed at which they do things, even the sparkle in their eyes. There is a noticeable difference, and perhaps understandably more so, with teens that were previously not feeling connected to their purpose that recently have begun to feel connected. Indeed, this is one way to encourage purpose, which leads to an overall sense of health and happiness. In the recommendations section, I share some thoughts from teens and how to support this connection.

Focus/Commitment

In addition to connection and personal meaning, teens found that both focus and commitment are important foundations for purpose. I include both in this section, since I have found that focus and commitment are closely related. While not impossible, it is difficult to have focus without some sort of commitment.

Sitting around a campfire one night with a small group of teens and adults, the conversation arose around focus and commitment being a necessary part of purpose. As we talked, one idea that emerged was that when one has purpose, it leads to commitment, which, in turn, gives you focus. In other words, if you really want to do something or have that deep feeling of needing to do it, you will be committed and focused.

The question was also raised about whether it was possible to be overly focused. We tossed this one around for a while, and in the end, it was decided that being overly focused can be both good and bad. As an example of the ups and downs of overfocusing, musicians or athletes who practice for hours and hours every day but who have gone off the rails were brought up.

Focus and commitment are indeed related to purpose. It would be easy to say that in order to have purpose, you must have focus and commitment. You can't really have purpose without commitment and along with that comes focus. In this small group, we agreed that your purpose will fuel your commitment and it's also true that your purpose needs to be fed with your commitment and your focus. We also agreed that it can be all too easy to get derailed from your purpose.

Life deals us many important and seemingly important sidetracks that need attention or get attention and this may move teens away from their purpose. For teens, there may be even more sidetracks to take or perhaps they are not yet used to dealing with the sidetracks the way adults are. Focus and commitment are important for a teen's life purpose to be fully realized.

So What Do We Do Now?

We all have the need for purpose. I have been asked many times about whether I think teens actually need purpose, suggesting that is something that comes later in life and is not necessary before then. My answer is simply that, yes, teens need purpose. Purpose actually starts at an early age. Now this may not be one's life purpose, but certainly, it is purpose; the why is there.

What if teens lack purpose? In the recommendations section, I provide some examples of how to support teen purpose. If you feel that the teens in your life lack purpose, then it is a good time to take pause and look deeper into what is happening. Are they really lacking purpose or is their ability to live that purpose blocked somehow?

As adults, we sometimes have a hard time spotting teen purpose and it gets even harder when a teen's natural tendency towards novelty or new experiences gives the appearance of lacking purpose and focus. Teens can focus on many things even when it seems they bounce from one activity to another or one area of interest to another. Their focus can be pretty intense and long lasting. It's a matter of cultivating it and making space for it to flourish. We adults can support teens in finding and living their purpose.

Like we have been doing throughout this book, we will use questions to help with reflection. In the event that you aren't reading this book chapter by chapter, I have been providing some suggestions about how to approach answering these questions.

Of course, you do not have to use any of them. These questions are not about a right or wrong answer. Don't worry about what you think the answers are supposed to be; just answer as honestly as you can. It's about bringing awareness to what is happening and having time for reflection. You may find that just answering these questions provides new insight or a new perspective.

So whether you're a teen or adult reading this book, the questions are here to get you to think about teen purpose. If you're an adult that isn't a parent to teens but works with teens, answer the questions based on what you have observed from working with teens.

As with all the questions in this book, grab a piece of paper and a pen, get comfortable, sit back, relax and have fun answering the following questions:

- *Question 1:* From what you know about purpose, would you say the teen/s in your life has/have purpose? Why?
- *Question 2:* Describe how the teen/s in your life exhibits/exhibit purpose.
- *Question 3:* What is personally meaningful to the teen/s in your life? How do you know?
- *Question 4:* What does/do the teen/s in your life feel connected to? What do they do without any thought of rewards or accolades?
- *Question 5:* What are the obstacles to the teen/s in your life having purpose? What is keeping him/her from connecting with something bigger than themselves with focus and commitment?

As with all the questions in this book, I suggest revisiting these questions from time to time to note any changes and to see your progress. These questions are a guide to exploration and I invite you to come up with your own.

I offer the following recommendations for purpose based on my work with teens in the field that will offer some insight into the above questions.

Encourage Teens To Engage In Something Meaningful

When teens are searching for purpose, and even when they have found it, adults can be instrumental by encouraging teens to engage in something meaningful. Adults all too often worry that if teens do this, they may have less time to engage in things like school studies, chores, etc.

We don't necessarily want to encourage teens to shun everything else in their life besides their purpose, though there is time for both. And if adults encourage teens, they can help them find the connection between their purpose and other activities that perhaps seem unrelated. This happens when adults treat what is meaningful to teens seriously, as they encourage them to make it a part of their life. I do hear a lot from adults that some teens have very little that is meaningful to them. Even if this is the case, they still have something or a few things that are meaningful to them and that is where the focus needs to be.

One way to encourage teens to pursue something meaningful is for adults to engage in something that is meaningful to them. In this way, there is common ground and experience to share. Not only will this help the teen feel connected with the adult, it will help them feel like they are not alone in these pursuits.

15-year-old Alex told me that he always felt that his grandfather encouraged him to spend time on what he found meaning in. He said that he and his grandfather would talk about both of their lives, with his grandfather sharing his stories about what he used to and still found meaning and importance in. Alex believed that this was a big part of why he spent time on

133

what was meaningful for him. "My grandfather showed me that it was okay and good to do the things that mean something to you. He has a pretty good life. I think its because he does what's important to him and doesn't worry much about other things."

Having Various Experiences

As has been noted, teens' interests will probably vary and change with time. Trying various activities, especially early in the teen years, can help teens figure out what their purpose is and even what they are passionate about. Sometimes purpose is already there without having to try many things or engage in various activities. I submit then that when teens engage with the world in various ways, it enhances their purpose; it doesn't take away from it.

Adults have asked whether it can be harmful for teens to try so many different activities and not really give full attention to one or two. Generally, there is no harm in this, though it might make for a busy, hectic schedule. However, if this becomes an established pattern over an extended period of time, it might be an indication that the teen has some fears around failure.

As teens engage with different aspects of the world by trying out new things, they have experiences. Experience does a lot for teens in that it gives them a foundation and something to work from. When teens have varied experiences, it is likely to bring them out of their comfort zone, which can actually help them become more aligned with their purpose. We all have had the experience of how being out of our comfort zone leads to self-growth and new interests and this is indeed true and important for teens.

Joy, a high school senior, shared her thoughts with me on this. "The more things I am able to try, the more I learn. Sometimes I realize that I

134

enjoy something more than I thought I would and sometimes it's the opposite; I thought I would like it or wasn't sure and I found out that I don't really. Maybe it didn't help me find my purpose, but it did help me know what my purpose isn't."

Be supportive when teens want to have various experiences, as it will help them find or solidify their purpose. Try not to project your fears unto teens and honestly consider their requests for experiences.

It's A Journey

Living one's purpose really is a lifelong journey. You can know your purpose and still it will manifest in different ways over time. For example, if a teen knows that her purpose is to work with disadvantaged youth, there are many ways to do that. So her purpose would stay the same, but how it manifests might change. She may, for instance, start out in one area of focus in working with disadvantaged youth, but years later may end up in another for any number of reasons.

For teens, having adults around them who know, understand, and to some degree, have experienced this is important in helping them work to understand this in their own way. So many teens feel that they are supposed to have this all figured out with an exact road map to what their life is going to look like. In some respects, it's a notion that they pick up from society, though that does seem to be becoming less so as our society recognizes its own shifts. The days of staying with the same job, doing the exact same thing for 30 to 40 years, while they maybe are not completely gone, are dwindling.

Part of the journey has to include time for reflection. Reflection or reflective practice is a foundational piece of the journey. It's important in the evolution of the journey and helping to ascertain whether the journey is still on track, even though it may change. There are a host of ways to be reflective or to have a reflective practice. I can't say that any one way is best though. It's truly about making the time and having it become a lifestyle.

Teens want to know that living their purpose is a lifetime journey and that they don't really need to have it all figured out at 18. Frank, a 17-year-old on his way to college, said, "It makes everything easier when you realize that even when you know what you want to do, it may not look exactly the way you thought it would and that's okay."

Passion

If purpose is the reason for doing something, then passion is the feeling one has about doing it. And while it is being done, passion doesn't always have to be related to a teen's life purpose. Many experts say that passion changes, so in reality, a teen can be passionate about many things and, in my experience, they often are.

So if passion changes, teens can be excited or feel passionate about a new experience or something they would like to do. This is, indeed, wonderful and should be encouraged. It's likely that a teen will be passionate about something for a certain duration of time and then will no longer be passionate or as passionate about it as they once were. There is no need to worry, as this is a natural part of being a teen and their search for novelty. Sometimes adults view this as being fickle or frivolous. I say, as long as teens are passionate about what they are doing in general, it is a good thing. Imagine a teen not being passionate about anything; that can be a cause for concern.

With teens, passion and purpose are related, in that when teens are engaged in their purpose, they are usually passionate about it. As mentioned above, with other endeavors teens may feel passionate about them at the time or for a fixed period of time and thereafter the passion wanes. Sadly, I do believe that the passions of many teens often get squashed for reasons mentioned above and also because they are expected to follow a prescriptive way of learning and being.

Adults should do their level best to nurture teens' passions so that they lead to a lifetime of passion and curiosity. As I always say, if you can't do that, at least don't get in the way. And if you suddenly realize you are in the way, then do what you can to get out of the way. Please don't misunderstand me. I firmly believe that teens need adults in their lives. In fact, I think this helps teens develop passion. We do know that at times adults knowingly and unknowingly can be a barrier to this development.

As in the previous chapters, I go right into the questions, recommendations and examples since they will provide enough of a framework to understand the nuances of passion.

So What Do We Do Now?

Passion is how we feel about what we are engaging in. We know that teens have passion. Teen passion needs to be nurtured and supported so that at the very least they can enjoy the feeling of being excited or passionate about what they are doing. Yes, teens can have many passions and these can change. This wonderful time where one can have so many passions should be embraced and celebrated.

It's true that along with this intense passion comes intense emotion and some would say you can't have one without the other. For the most part, my experience has shown that teens' passion and emotion are tied together. When there is passion, usually there's an emotional investment, even if it's for a short time. Adults don't necessarily need to do anything with that other than to be supportive and understanding. I know that teens respond well when adults support and are understanding towards their passions. As mentioned above, these passions may take precedence for teens, even when adults wish they wouldn't.

Most adults want the teens in their life to be healthy and happy and don't want to stand in the way when teens feel passion for something. It can be difficult when adults feel that a teen might be headed down a bumpy or risky road. As adults, the best we can do is continue to be a part of the process with teens and let their passions take them down the bumpy roads and even the risky ones, provided that they do not put the teen's life or the lives of others in danger. Teens will learn a lot from the bumpy roads.

Like we have been doing throughout this book, we will use questions to help with reflection. In the event that you aren't reading this book chapter by chapter, I have been providing some suggestions about how to approach answering these questions.

Of course, you do not have to use any of them. These questions are not about a right or wrong answer. Don't worry about what you think the answers are supposed to be; just answer as honestly as you can. It's about bringing awareness to what is happening and having time for reflection. You may find that just answering these questions provides new insight or a new perspective.

So whether you're a teen or adult reading this book, the questions are here to get you to think about teen passion. If you're an adult that isn't a parent to teens but works with teens, answer the questions based on what you have observed from working with teens.

As with all the questions in this book, grab a piece of paper and a pen, get comfortable, sit back, relax and have fun answering the following questions:

- *Question 1:* What is/are the teen/s in your life passionate about right now?
- *Question 2:* Describe how you know when the teen/s in your life is/are passionate about something.
- *Question 3:* In general, would you say that the teen/s in your life is/are passionate?
- *Question 4:* In what ways do you support the teen/s in your life's passions? How often do you talk to him/her about what they are currently passionate about?
- *Question 5:* In general, do teens have enough time to follow their passions? What gets in the way of this happening?

As with all the questions in this book, I suggest revisiting these questions from time to time to note any changes and to see your progress. These questions are a guide to exploration and I invite you to come up with your own.

I offer the following recommendations for nurturing teen passion based on my work with teens in the field that will offer some insight into the above questions.

If Passion Exists, Support It

Do the very best you can to support teens' passions. You don't necessarily have to change your whole life around in order to do this. It's about making time and space and being open to figuring out ways to allow teens to pursue their passions. As has been noted, teens' passions can change with time, so it may not be practical or prudent to invest in every passion a teen may have. With the ones that stick, the ones the teen keeps going back to and have had as a passion for a while, maybe even years, those are the ones you can invest in.

Being supportive doesn't always mean you like or understand why your teen has a particular passion. Your teen can be passionate about something that you find boring or lacking stimulation. Do your best to be supportive anyway and try to find out what you can about their passion by talking with them about it. It's okay to say to teens something like, 'I don't really share your passion for this, but I do want to support you.' Even if you don't know exactly how to support them, just being committed to it will present opportunities.

Just as important is that adults have the power to take away teens' passion by not being supportive and by not being willing to have conversations about it. I am reminded of a conversation I had with Andre, who was in his first year of college. "I think I had a lot of passions and now I have less. I don't think my parents knew how to support me or maybe they thought they had to be perfect or know a lot about what I was passionate about. I was lucky, I think, because if I was doing something at school, they usually didn't think about it too much. I used time during and after school to follow my passions. Adults can help just by giving the support that they can."

Let Passion Develop

When adults share their passions with teens, it can be wonderful. When adults share their passions with teens expecting them to have the same passions, it can be detrimental. There's no time frame or correct number of passions a teen should have. In the same way, there isn't a right way to have passion. As adults, we can relax a little bit in knowing that we can let passion develop in teens. Yes, adults sometimes worry if they feel the teens in their life don't have passions. We have to let passion develop and we can help by creating opportunities for teens.

There are some who say the whole need for passion thing is exaggerated. Sure, that idea may have some merit when it comes to having one particular passion. It may not be necessary to have just one thing you're passionate about or to follow it to the ends of the earth. However, passion and curiosity are related, so while we don't want to panic if it seems teens do not have any passion, we also want to recognize that passion does have a place in teen health and happiness. Since passion is more about the feeling we get when engaged or looking forward to engaging in something, it's important that this excitement is nourished in teens. It's a good thing to feel excitement and have passion.

One of the most profound statements I have heard from a teen was when Rebecca, a high school senior, was talking to our group about passion. "You don't always have to have passion for everything. You may not be able to do your passions all the time, but having passions is what makes life interesting. It might take a long time to find even one thing you're passionate about or you might have a lot you're passionate about; either way works. That's what I've noticed."

Learning About Passions

When teens have real opportunities to learn about their passions, it is one of the best ways to keep particular passions and the idea of passions alive. This doesn't mean that adults have to heavily invest in every single passion a teen has, but adults can help teens find places or people where they can learn more about their passion in real time.

One area that can be utilized at first is technology or the Internet. Most teens are pretty adept at using technology and the Internet to explore topics or interest areas. Initially, this can be used to learn more about their passions, which then will give teens a better idea of whether they want to continue to pursue that passion or not.

We will expand on learning in another chapter, so I will not go into great detail about technology and its role in learning. I'll share a brief thought here though: Technology does not and I believe will not ever replace learning in real time. For example, you can watch a video on how to change a tire, but until you do it or apply what you've learned, you haven't experienced what it feels like to actually do it.

It is important for teens to learn from someone who has practical experience with his or her passion. It doesn't have to be the exact same experience, though the closer you can get, the better. Sometimes a teen will spend time learning about a certain passion only to discover that they either want to focus on a specific area of that passion or something totally different.

Denise, who was working on her college applications, told me that because she took time to learn about her passions, she had a better idea of what she wanted to focus on. "I thank my parents for helping me find out more about my passions. Now I know what I want to focus on. Even though I still have other passions, I am more focused."

Chapter Nine

Empowerment & Voice

Two hot topics of late are teen empowerment and voice. You may have heard this in reference to student voice and empowerment or youth voice and empowerment. Teens need to have a voice. They need to have a say in what's happening to them. They often see and have to figure out decisions that are made about them, for them and around them by adults.

Having a say in issues or decisions that affect you is about having real input and making a contribution to the process. Teens should be afforded this fundamental right. I do get pushback from adults on this point often, as they feel teens should not have any say in important decisions. They will cleverly use my statements that teens can be impulsive and tend towards novelty against me and suggest this is the reason they are against teens having a voice. Teens having a voice is about them being taken seriously and being able to voice their feelings, concerns, thoughts and ideas.

To this point in the book I have been an advocate for both teens and adults, suggesting the importance of adults and teens coming together for teen health and happiness. This still holds true. When it comes to teen voice, too many adults misinterpret it to mean an iteration of "Lord of the Flies." Teen voice is not always the absence of adult voice. In my work with teens, when teens have real voice, it is in partnership with adults. Since it is a very different exchange than the norm, teens seek adult input.

What I have come to realize is adults who are uncomfortable with teen voice either have never experienced it or have experienced it in a way that was about elevating one voice over another. So it makes sense that some adults are uncomfortable with teen voice and even more uncomfortable with teen empowerment.

A number of my friends and colleagues who work with teen voice and empowerment not only make a distinction between voice and empowerment, but they treat them separately. As we will see in a moment, they are different and yet connected. Because I ultimately want to see teens being empowered to be the masters of their health and happiness, I see voice and empowerment as belonging to the same whole. My colleagues and friends who do it differently have their own ironclad reasons for doing so and are just as effective. I invite you to look at the good work that is out there on youth voice and empowerment.

Empowerment, as I have to come to understand it within the context of my work, is a process in which teens have more control over or become the masters of their health, happiness, and ultimately, their lives. The idea is that teens have a path to self-knowledge through empowerment. While we can never really empower another, we can support them in empowering themselves. To me, voice is a way to empowerment, as fully and honestly expressing oneself begins with having a voice.

For the remainder of this chapter I will discuss voice and empowerment together and will use recommendations and examples to illustrate their connection. What follows are the foundations of voice and empowerment shared with me by teenagers, along with some observations of my own. These are shared within the context of teen health and happiness.

Expression

To fully and honestly express oneself is one of life's real challenges. The truth is that it may be something we continuously strive for. Teens spend a good deal of time trying to figure out what they want to express and how to express it. They do come up against a societal system that devalues this sort of expression in general and for them specifically.

I can tell you that I have many adults who tell me that teens nowadays are overly encouraged to express themselves. There may be some truth to this; however, I have come to feel that this sentiment has more to do with what adults see as a lack of teen resilience rather than truly having too many ways to honestly express themselves. If we stop and think about the life of a teen today, we will recognize that today's teens are watched, listened in on and regulated to an unprecedented degree. To be sure, they have myriad ways of communicating and expressing themselves thanks to technology, and with the way technology is watched, their expression a lot of the times isn't always authentic.

Even if teens do have ways to fully and honestly express themselves with each other, they don't have them when it involves adults. In this type of expression, adults do not need to approve of it or even accept it, so adults don't get to say what is valid and what isn't.

Without this true expression, teens' voice and empowerment are not possible. I haven't witnessed any instances when teen expression was shut down that led to them having a real voice and being truly empowered. We know that shutting down expression also has a negative impact on teen health and happiness.

Teens feel empowered and like they have voice when they can actively participate in their own lives. Teens need to be involved in decisions that impact them in the immediate and long term. You may find as an adult that teens aren't always interested in participating in every single decision or issue that arises even when you feel they should. What you will also find is that the more empowered they feel and the more they feel like they have voice, the more involved they will be. Teens participating in their health and happiness looks a lot like being involved in the process and having access to it. It's difficult to be involved in the process if you don't have access to it.

Teen involvement requires a commitment from both teens and adults to a process of inclusion, as well as trust and honest sharing of information. The common criticism from today's adults with regard to a lack of teen involvement — from civics to anything that adults deem important — is in part because teens do not have access to this type of involvement and/or are not included. Teens are excluded on purpose or because no one thought to invite them. In either case, they aren't there.

It's increasingly apparent that teens need to be involved in the decisions, issues and actions that affect them. When they are involved, they develop an understanding of the variables that impact their options. Teens even develop an understanding of what adults have to consider when making decisions or taking action.

A common question is whether teens should be involved to the fullest extent, especially when it comes to more serious matters or ones in which adults feel they should be protected from. Some adults feel we should let teens still have that innocence of the teen years. Teens know a lot about the world and they know the world isn't always a happy place.

When it comes to decisions and issues that affect their health and happiness, we should always strive to be honest with teens. We should ensure that they can participate in what affects them. And when we have an honest, inclusive process in place, it will become clear what to do in these dilemmas.

For parents, you needn't have a formalized process in place, though it can help to have agreements or a way of doing things. For adults who work with teens, a more formalized process is best.

Balance Of Power

In order for empowerment and voice to be authentic, there has to be a balance of power between adults and teens. This means the power to make decisions and act has to be equitable and that this balance should not be skewed in the adult's favor. I want to be clear when I say this that I am referring to decisions that impact teens' health and happiness. If a decision needs to be made about home finances or something of a similar ilk, it would be great if a parent or guardian decides to include teens, but it's not critical.

Adults that work with teens need to ensure that teens have an equal voice and equal ways to have control over their lives. For instance, if you include teens on a school committee along with adults, make sure you have as many teens on that committee as adults or even more teens than adults. If this can't happen, make sure teen representation holds the same weight as adult representation; otherwise, it's just an exercise. There has to be equity in power because without it an unequal power relationship exists.

So What Do We Do Now?

Teens have power and voice and we need to nurture this so they know about themselves and what is best for their health and happiness. We can't empower anyone, but we can create the conditions and opportunities for them to empower themselves. Using their power and their voice, teens will have choices for their life that will allow them to have a say in what happens to them. In this way, teens gain the knowledge to make decisions that work best for them.

When teens are empowered, they are free to expand their understanding and the control they have over various aspects of their lives. Teen voice and empowerment break down barriers between teens and adults. When teens are empowered, the difference in their relationship with adults compared to when they don't feel empowered is vast.

Sometimes when adults hear phrases like 'teen empowerment' or 'teen voice', they envision teens having full choice and that no adult input is ever considered. This is not the case. Teen voice and empowerment can happen without adult input or scrutiny; just as often, it happens in conjunction with adults. In a very real sense, teen empowerment and voice, if authentic, comes into contact with the adult world. When teens are empowered to the point that they are the masters of their own lives, they will be engaging with adults and their peers.

Ultimately, voice and empowerment are processes that continue throughout a lifetime that allow teens to have the power to participate fully in their own lives and the world at large. In this way, they make decisions and take action on things that are important to them.

In most of the chapters, we have been using questions to help with reflection. In the same spirit, we will continue to do so in this chapter.

Of course, you do not have to use any of the questions. These questions are not about a right or wrong answer. Don't worry about what you think the answers are supposed to be; just answer as honestly as you can. These questions are designed to get you to reflect and think about teen voice and empowerment. You may find that just answering these questions provides new insight or a new perspective.

So whether you're a teen or adult reading this book, the questions are here to get you to think about teen empowerment and voice. If you're an adult that isn't a parent to teens but works with teens, answer the questions based on what you have observed from working with teens.

As with all the questions in this book, grab a piece of paper and a pen, get comfortable, sit back, relax and have fun answering the following questions:

- *Question 1:* Does/do the teen/s in your life have the freedom to express him/herself/themselves? Is his or her/Are their voice/s taken as seriously as adults? How do you think the teen/s in your life would answer this question?

- *Question 2:* How would you characterize the teen/s in your life's empowerment? Is he or she/Are they empowered to make decisions about his or her/their lives without adult interference?

- *Question 3:* How often do you and the teen/s in your life collaborate where their input holds the same weight as yours?

- *Question 4:* In what ways do you make space and provide opportunities for teens to empower themselves?

- *Question 5:* What are the barriers for the teen/s in your life to become fully empowered?

As with all the questions in this book, I suggest revisiting these questions from time to time to note any changes and to see your progress. These questions are a guide to exploration and I invite you to come up with your own.

The words and thoughts of teens will shape the following recommendations and examples of teen empowerment and voice. I have had the pleasure in working with teens to elevate their voice and empower them. I will add some of my insights as well, but will do so sparingly in this section.

Recommendations/Examples

Taking Action

Adults can support teens in empowering themselves if they can help teens take action. Voice and empowerment take hold when they are put into action. Adults have to understand that without this, teens would just be going through the motions and perhaps voicing their concerns and ideas, but never truly exercising their power and agency to take charge of their health and happiness.

There are many ways for teens to take action. The action taken is best if it arises from something that teens are authentically interested in that affects them directly. Since this book is about teen health and happiness, there are actions teens can take that will enhance their health and happiness. Many of the areas and types of actions they can take are discussed throughout this book. There isn't necessarily one action that is better than another. So long as the action being taken is truly coming from the teen, then it is empowering.

The more impactful the action, the more empowered teens will become. It's important for adults to let teens take action, to support it when and if they can and to be really interested in it. Teens thrive when they can take action that impacts their health and happiness.

Noah, who was 16 at the time, explained it to a group of teens and adults in this way: "Anytime I can take real action that actually is about my health, it feels good, like I have some control. I can be responsible for myself and not always have to rely on adults." Undoubtedly, this does not only apply in areas that would be considered health and happiness but to any action.

Making Real Choices

One of the biggest mistakes I have witnessed when it comes to teen voice and empowerment is to only give teens the ability to make menial choices; choices that don't have any impact or are not really choices because they have to be agreed upon by adults. My best words of advice are, don't pretend that teens have the ability to make real choices when they don't. They can sniff that out pretty quickly and trust will diminish. Be honest about the choices that they do have, for instance, with respect to health. In most places in the world, teens cannot make medical decisions until they reach the legal age of adulthood. As adults, we need to be honest with teens about this and also hear their thoughts and concerns.

I, for one, am a big advocate for allowing teens to make their own choices in a general sense and specifically when it comes to their health and happiness. There's no question that teens sometimes do not make good choices when it comes to their health and happiness. The reality is they will probably find a way to make bad choices anyway. If they feel they do not have to hide these choices from adults, it at least opens up avenues of communication. The bad choices are about just having the ability to make a real choice because they haven't had opportunities to make choices. Though I have written this earlier, it's worth repeating. If we want teens to make good choices, then we have to give them the opportunity to make and process them.

While teens cannot make medical decisions, they can certainly make decisions regarding their nutrition, forms of exercise, self-expression and so on. Teens appreciate having these real choices, especially when it comes about from honest discovery alongside adults.

Jill, a high school student who was going into her senior year in high school, told me that the more opportunities she had to make choices about her health and happiness, the more she made the 'right' choices. "You know, Peter, I think that because I was able to make choices I didn't have to sneak around or try to hide something. I knew that making a bad choice wouldn't be a good idea. Because I am the one making the choices, I also have to be the one who is responsible for them."

Solving Real-World Problems

This may seem out of place in a book about teen health and happiness. What does solving real-world problems have to do with teen health and happiness? It has a lot to do with it in the context of voice and empowerment. In order for teens to be truly happy and healthy, they have to have a real voice and empower themselves to be the masters of their own lives. Having teens solve real-world problems will do this. The problems can have a wide range, so long as they are real and the solutions teens come up with and the actions they take are acted upon in a serious manner.

There are plenty of real-world problems that directly and indirectly impact teen health and happiness. If there are some that arise that you feel fall outside this scope, this is okay. In fact, it's a good thing. Don't worry so much about fitting the problems into a specific category so long as they are real. One example from teens that I worked with from a town school was the lack of access to healthy school lunches. This was a real-world problem with some simple and not-so-simple solutions. The key was to ensure that what the teens proposed would be given serious consideration and that their actions were not fruitless. We all know that sometimes, despite the best proposals and plan of action, nothing or very little happens. This is okay as a lesson, but it doesn't mean teens have to stop working on the problem.

As I have said many times, teens are resilient and can be very persistent when they are passionate about an issue and see a way forward. Working on real-world problems comes with everything a real-world problem has to offer. Teens tend to feel good about their work even when it doesn't go their way. Sure, they may be disappointed and even frustrated, but they did have an opportunity to work on a real-world problem.

Dave, a freshman in college, was reflecting with me on his high school and first-year college experience. We talked about the opportunities he had to work on real-world problems. "We needed more opportunities to work on problems that were real and had meaning. When I had the chance to work on something real for my senior project, it showed me that I could do something worthwhile. I solved a problem for the community and that made

154

me feel like I was a part of the community, like I was able to give something back. Most of the things I did in school weren't as real as that."

Solving real-world problems empowers teens and allows them to positively contribute, not only to their own health and happiness, but also to that of others.

Chapter Ten

Learning

Learning is a natural process that has been part of our existence since we were first considered modern-day humans in the Evolutionary Model, roughly 200,000 years ago, and roughly 10,000 years ago in the Creationist Model. Whichever view you subscribe to, the fact remains that humans have been around for a very long time without any form of 'compulsory' or 'formalized' schooling or education system. After all, learning is a natural process in human beings.

Just watch any infant and/or toddler and you will be amazed at how much and quickly they learn effortlessly. At this time, they are not in school, at least the way we think about it today. They learn what they want and when they want something. Some of you might be thinking, wait a minute, when my child was two, I taught her how to read or recognize shapes, etc. While this is true, it is more a reflection of the fact that the child wanted to learn and was curious to know what you know. As I am sure many of you can attest, if a child of this age is not willing or ready to learn something, it's not going to happen.

The question then becomes, without school, how did humans learn anything? How did they learn the things they needed to in order to survive and even thrive for so long without school? The simple answer to these and other related questions is that learning is natural. In fact, it is such a natural process that it is difficult to turn it off. Even the most passive mind is learning all the time. Whether the learning sticks is another matter.

Now, I can hear the gasps and see the raised eyebrows as some of you might be thinking, so if learning is so natural, then teachers and schools should have a very easy job and all of our schools should be places where everyone cannot wait to go to. As we all know, this is not the case. Compulsory schooling takes a very natural process and tries to force it into completely unnatural confines, constraints and narrow bandwidth. From this stems the very real consequences that teachers, schools, parents, students and our education system try to resolve on a daily basis.

What we have at the moment is a system that is designed to produce an uneducated, controllable mass workforce, combined with the natural process of learning being made unnatural and contrived. It makes sense, then, that for so many school is something to be avoided at all costs and is a source of frustration and angst.

It may sound like I am advocating for the abolishment of school as a whole. This is not the case. There are many wonderful things taking place in schools across the country, be they public, private, charter or otherwise. However, I am advocating for the transformation of our current education system so that it is in line with the fact that learning is natural and schooling is optional. Schooling and learning are not always the same thing. Unfortunately, many teens spend much of their day in schools or places where they should be free to learn but instead are subjected to practices that diminish their curiosity and will to learn.

I could fill the rest of this chapter with a description of the various practices in schools that I have found to be damaging and in direct opposition to the very real idea of humans and — in the context of this book — teens as natural learners. Rather than do that, I will direct you to a great article written by Jerry Mintz, the Executive Director of the Alternative Education Resource

Organization (AERO), entitled, "The Ten Signs You Need to Find a Different Kind of Education for Your Child." I provide a brief synopsis here.

If the teen or teens in your life are saying things like they hate school, if they dread going or come home complaining about conflicts they've had in school with adults or peers, these are signs that they need a different type of setting. Further, if they have lost interest in learning and creative expression and/or are always waiting until the last minute to do their homework, if they have problems communicating with adults or if you have adults at the school that suggest that your teen has any number of various disorders, it may be time to find a different kind of setting.

I will add a note here about school start times for teens. In brief, school start times should be after 9 am for optimal cognitive functioning for teens, among many other benefits. I will offer my thoughts on this subject in the chapter on sleep.

Learning is such a natural process that it doesn't need to be forced. It may require guidance, but not force. Learning is essential to teen health and happiness for without it there is little left but repetition. Teens want to and need to learn. As mentioned in a previous chapter, they do have a propensity to seek novelty and move through various interests, passions and activities and this is, in large part, due to their natural curiosity and drive to learn.

I have been fortunate to have had many conversations with teens about learning. What I have shared below are the major themes from their thoughts, my observations and the implementation of practices that support and encourage learning.

Engaging the whole person or practicing a holistic brand of learning has to include the intellectual, social, emotional, physical and spiritual dimensions of a person; moreover, all of these elements need to be engaged for deep, personalized learning that stays with you to take place. Learning can take place without all of these aspects engaged. It's just that the learning will be different. It will tend to be surface learning or learning that is forgotten within a short amount of time. Many of my colleagues and friends in the field would make the argument that anything that is forgotten in a short amount of time isn't learning; it's merely short-term recall. I agree for the most part, though, I do think you can resurrect short-term recall in order to facilitate deep learning.

Teens today need learning that engages every aspect of who they are. It's clear that much of what is called or expected to be learning isn't really learning at all. While learning that engages the whole person can happen inside a 'classroom', it is more likely that it will happen outside of it. Teens need to be out in their community, learning with it and from it. In this way, they not only begin to know themselves better, they are part of the real, everyday life of the community.

There isn't much dispute in the research that deep learning is as much an emotional experience as an intellectual one. When a teen's heart, soul, mind and body are engaged, learning becomes internalized and a part of who they are. There is also significant research that tells us that movement and learning are connected. At some level, we need to physically engage with the learning. It doesn't have to be a complete kinesthetic experience where a teen must be moving all the time, though learning without any sort of movement is challenging.

If we accept the notion that we remember most what we are emotionally connected to, consider the impact of our souls being touched. When our souls are touched, we are capable of great acts of humanity, kindness, courage and growth. Certainly, not every learning experience will be that profound. What can happen is that learning is thought of as connecting a teen's mind, body and spirit.

We truly have a plethora of resources at our disposal, which teens and adults can take advantage of, that supports learning and engages the whole person.

Creativity

Sir Ken Robinson, a leading proponent of creativity, especially as it related to creativity in schools, suggests that creativity is a critical 21st century skill for solving our current and future issues. He further suggests that creativity is part of a process that may begin with a hunch or idea and is connected with critical thinking and evaluation. It's true that we are careening headlong into the unprecedented challenges of the 21st century. Creativity will be necessary to address these challenges in ways that are just and sustainable.

Anyone can be creative, and that may look different, depending on what is being engaged with and who is engaging. Having spent thousands of hours with teens, I can attest to the importance and uniqueness of creativity. Teens can be more creative than adults, even if some of their ideas are a bit grandiose. Creativity is an essential part of learning and is also an avenue for

160

expression and problem solving. We sometimes think of creativity as something reserved for artists or entertainers. To be sure, there is a good deal of creativity in these fields. Creativity is also about approaching things in a fresh, new way.

Teens are naturally inclined towards creativity and they tend to get steered away from creativity by well-meaning and not-so-well-meaning adults who see creativity as something superfluous. In our school system, which we have already established is often antithetical to creativity, much of it is deemphasized. It's about getting the right prescribed answer rather than a creative process of testing and evaluation.

Teens do need the time and space to be creative. If you have been around teens, you will see that. When they are moved by something, they will find creative ways to get involved with it. I have been inspired by the teens I have worked with. They have always made me be more creative, whether it's because of a deliberate challenge or because I had to step up my game in response to their feedback.

Creativity is important to learning and teen health and happiness. The easiest way to kill creativity is to hover, get overinvolved in the process and give unasked-for feedback and praise. The easiest way to support it is to give the time and space for teens to be creative.

Deep Understanding That Is Not Limited By Subject Areas

I have always had a fun a challenge when I start working with teens that helps them think about how learning is connected and not just about a subject area. I ask them to think of a subject, idea, object, discipline, etc., that is disconnected from everything else. For instance, is math really just math or

161

is it perhaps connected to other subject areas? I have received many outstanding answers over the years but none that weren't connected to something else. The idea behind this thought exercise is to emphasis how learning and knowledge don't happen in specific, unyielding categories. In fact, learning without understanding how it's connected is very limited.

For certain, we do have people who are experts in a particular area or vocation, and in that sense, it seems what they do is segmented into specific sets of skills and areas of knowledge. After all, a chef isn't laying a cement floor as s/he prepares meals. The chef knows much about food preparation and s/he also uses elements of math and science, at minimum, to prepare meals.

Deep understanding comes from discovering and uncovering the intricacies of what you're learning about. Teens have the capacity and want to do this. If you have ever observed a teen when they are given the time and space to go deeply into what they are doing, it's inspiring. This theme, as have the others, came from my conversations with teens and reflections on my own practices. Learning is really about following a path and understanding that subject areas such as math, science and history exist not to disconnect one from the other but to serve as a framework.

Teens can get confused when they see adults having certain professions and knowing a lot about that or other particular areas and seemingly little about others. Again, the idea is that what teens and adults do every day entails many different skillsets and understanding, even though there is a focus area.

Another point to make is that in the everyday world learning doesn't stop so that we can ring a bell or punch a clock. Learning must also be about application through experience. This is often referred to as experiential learning, where learning takes place through experience. In short, you learn by doing and reflecting on what you are doing. Through application and experience, learning is deeper and more meaningful. It's this type of learning that helps teens make long-lasting connections.

Looking at this from a brain-development or brain-mapping standpoint, new experiences form new neurological pathways in the brain and more areas of the brain are active during experiences and application, which, in turn, leads to deep understanding.

So What Do We Do Now?

Learning is human and perhaps what makes us human is our drive to learn. Any interaction between two or more human beings brings with it emotional, social, physical, spiritual and intellectual aspects. It doesn't just engage these areas but embraces them, sometimes by the simplest of human interactions. Pursuing knowledge together, inviting each other to learn and arousing each other's curiosity are tied to emotions and feelings. Real education goes beyond the acquisition of skills or knowledge. It gets to the heart of social relationships and ultimately what it means to be human.

Learning is integrated and the idea of learning rather than being limited by trying to name which style or philosophy is best would do well to take a page from integrative medicine. The idea behind any type of integration is one of embracing the exploration of all ideas that make sense and have the potential to be successful. Just as integrative medicine seeks to capitalize on the knowledge and experience of different 'approaches to health, wellness and medicine' (some stretching back thousands of years), weaving them together so that individuals can experience vibrant health, so too can education capitalize on the many different approaches to learning (some stretching back thousands of years), so that learning is a vibrant, beautifully-blended, internalized and personalized tapestry.

Learning has been and continues to be vigorously studied and hotly contested. Perhaps no other field is subject to so many proposed changes, gimmick programs, shotgun strategies and steadfast adherence to damaging practices all in the name of progression. There are various interests competing for attention, time and a financial inroad into the field of education. From the freelancers and consultants, to the private corporations with their replication models, there is no dearth of 'expert' ideas on how to best promote "learning', whatever the motivation may be.

We know that learning and schooling are not always the same thing; too often they are not. Teens can be engaged in meaningful learning that engages every aspect of who they are, allows for creativity and goes beyond limiting the learning by trying to classify it.

In previous chapters, we have been using questions to help with reflection. Below are some questions to help with that process.

Of course, you do not have to use any of the questions. These questions are not about a right or wrong answer. Don't worry about what you think the answers are supposed to be; just answer as honestly as you can. These questions are designed to get you to reflect and think about learning. You may find that just answering these questions provides new insight or a new perspective. So whether you're a teen or adult reading this book, the questions are here to get you to think about learning.

As with all the questions in this book, grab a piece of paper and a pen, get comfortable, sit back, relax and have fun answering the following questions:

- *Question 1:* How does/do the teen/s in your life feel about learning? What kind of things do they say when it comes to learning?
- *Question 2:* What words would you use to describe most of the teen/s in your life's learning? What are his/her pursuits of learning like?
- *Question 3:* Using the criteria so far in this chapter, what would you like to change about the learning the teen/s in your life engages/engage in?
- *Question 4:* Does/do the teen/s in your life get to see you learning or being creative?
- *Question 5:* Do you make space for the teen/s in your life to learn in a way that engages all aspects of who they are, allows for creativity and is geared towards deep understanding? What obstacles get in the way of this?

As with all the questions in this book, I suggest revisiting these questions from time to time to note any changes and to see your progress. These questions are a guide to exploration and I invite you to come up with your own.

The following recommendations and examples are taken directly from the thoughts shared with me by teens and my own observations and practices. Just like with all the recommendations and examples in this book, they are not meant to be comprehensive. They are the major, relevant themes that have come from my work.

Importance Of Finding The Right Learning Environment — The Right Fit

This chapter focused on what learning can look like for teens. An important theme that has come from my work with teens is the importance of the right fit with the learning environment. This is particularly important if the teen is enrolled in school, no matter the type, focus or size. Adults see this too in their professional environment. Some positions and organizations are the right fit, while others aren't. When it's the right fit, teens will thrive in their learning; when it isn't, they will struggle.

It would be difficult for me to put a number on how often I have seen a shift take place in students when they find the right environment. I have also been witness to the reverse happening where, for some reason, a student is no longer in an environment that was the right fit. The difference with either is staggering.

Rodney, who was ready to go into his first year of college, shared his experience with me. "I went to a school that I didn't like at all for about five years. I had friends and all, but I didn't connect with any of the teachers. I don't remember them being mean to me or any more mean to me than other kids. It just didn't feel right being there. I didn't do well there. I felt like I didn't know anything. The teachers made me feel like I was stupid. I don't think they yelled at me, but I could tell they thought I was dumb. I couldn't wait to leave there every day and never wanted to go back. It drove my parents crazy."

We talked a bit more about this and he told me that he was basically depressed while he was there. I asked what happened after those five years.

166

"My parents decided they would try homeschooling me. I went to our neighbors down the road because they homeschooled their kids too. It felt like a big relief. I could really learn about anything I wanted to. We did a lot of cool projects and we learned from each other. I felt smart again. After a couple of years, I decided to go back to a different school that I loved. The difference was almost night and day."

Justine and her parents came to me one day and explained the terrible time she was having in school. In short, the school was not a good fit for Justine for a variety of reasons; one of which is that the learning philosophy was more teacher-centered and passive. Justine presented with low energy and a palpable feeling of frustration and disenchantment with learning. After having a few more meetings, we started to search for an alternative. Eventually, Justine and her parents found the right fit. A few months after being in the new learning environment, Justine seemed to be a different person. She was vibrant, full of life and spoke to with joy and excitement about the various things she was working on.

The right learning environment doesn't have to be a school. It could be many other alternatives to traditional schooling. The key for adults is to be open to helping teens find the right fit. If that can't happen in school, then at the very least it can happen somewhere else. Taking the time to find the right learning environment can make a significant difference in teen health and happiness.

Meaningful Learning Based On Interests

Having the freedom to explore interests and go deeper into those areas of interest is what creates the opportunities for meaningful learning.

167

Many have written about and have explored the fact that when students are working on topics that interest them and have meaning, they will learn the three R's and many other important skills. In fact, this type of learning is more profound, longer lasting and makes it more likely that there is a personal investment in learning. The research is clear that when people of any age are working within an area of interest, they are more driven and productive. It isn't so much about not having tolerance for mundane tasks, it's about having a low threshold for doing things that others tell you have meaning when they really don't or they don't for you.

Teens understand that they have to trust the notion that sometimes the meaning in what they're doing isn't immediately apparent. They accept that. What they don't accept is when everything they do is a wait-and-see exercise; 'just wait, when you get older, you'll see how taking all these tests are meaningful.'

Meaningful learning can be a true partnership between adults and teenagers, where knowledge is shared and built upon. When it comes to meaningful learning, we have to listen to teens more often, trust them to make good decisions and make sure there is the freedom to explore interests and ideas so they can 'feel the learning'. Learning based on interests is certainly not a new idea. It's practiced in many places. Some adults question whether learning has to be solely based on interests. In my experience, this will make the learning more personalized and internalized.

Another question is about whether teens learning about only what they're interested in is limiting or leaves them lacking in skills. I have seen no evidence of this. The truth is that everyone has gaps in their knowledge; particular areas that come too easily and ones that we struggle with. Teens want to be involved in meaningful learning that stems from their interests.

I can remember having a conversation with the same group of teens on multiple occasions about learning based on interests and having meaning. "I don't understand why we are forced to learn things we are not interested in. We can learn so much more when we're interested in something. My father always tells me that sometimes you have to do things you don't want to do like pay bills or write checks. I get that. And when you do those things, you know there is a reason even if you don't like it. When I am interested in something, I usually can understand it and I can find the meaning in it. We know that everything isn't always going to be fun, but doing things just to do them is pointless."

Adults can advocate for learning that is meaningful and based on teen interests. In general, teens have multiple interests, so designing learning around these interests will be challenging and rewarding. Adults can also support teens in their pursuit of interest-based, meaningful learning by carving out time for it and encouraging teens to follow through with it.

Learning With And From The Community

In Chapter Nine, I wrote about how solving real-world problems is important in developing passion. Here we will discuss learning with and from the community.

Most communities are a treasure trove of knowledge waiting to be discovered and shared. I have found that most communities are very responsive and excited when it comes to helping teens learn. Community-based learning also has the added benefit of helping teens feel connected to their surroundings. As such, they tend to care more about their local community and will seek out the learning resources.

We know that with technology teens can seek out knowledge from their computers or mobile devices and they don't need to go into the community. Learning from the community will likely have a unique twist that you can't get anywhere else, plus that added layer of familiarity helps to bring learning into context.

In my opinion, teens need to be out learning from their and with their community. This ties in nicely with learning that engages the whole person, is meaningful, based on interests and it not limited by subject areas. When I had teens out in their community learning from it and with it, their investment in learning grew and they were usually surprised to find out that they lived in or near a community with such great resources.

We have this notion that we must go far and wide to learn. Sure, it's true that learning outside of our community also has tremendous benefits; however, teens don't always need to go far and wide to learn. In fact, it's been my experience that when teens are first learning from and with their community, they are more ready to reap the benefits of learning beyond it. They now have a comparison. Teens often find out a lot about their community and may develop new interests or passions because of it.

Tina, a tenth-grader, presented on her community-based learning experiences: "I never knew my community had all these things going on and so much I could learn from. There are a lot of people I can learn from too that I never knew were there. I found out that there are some big issues that people in the community have to deal with. I might be able to help."

Adults can help teens discover community resources and encourage teens to learn from and with them. If adults don't know about community resources, they can learn about them alongside teens. What a great model for teens to see.

Chapter Eleven

Gratitude & Respect

Gratitude and respect occupy a large space with regard to teen health and happiness. Teens get a bad rap when it comes to gratitude and respect. They are viewed as possessing little of either by many. The thing is that teens want and need both, especially respect.

Gratitude and respect are tied tightly together. You can have one without the other, as in, you can respect a person but not be grateful to have them in your life. In order for both of these to flourish, they need to work in tandem. Let me explain. There are a lot of prevailing thoughts on gratitude. What I have observed is that gratitude is about a way of being or a mindset of appreciation. It's also about being grateful or feeling the emotion of gratitude. It shows in your thoughts and actions; perhaps most noticeable in the way you go about caring for yourself and others.

There are thoughts about respect in our culture as well. We tend to focus on respect between people. What I have noticed is that respect is about how we treat everything. We may have respect because we have admiration for someone or an appreciation for a set of ideas and behaviors. For instance, we can appreciate the work of a car mechanic or admire someone for how they treat people or what they were able to accomplish. It's true that you can have respect for people but not respect someone's possessions or what we consider to be the natural world. What is also true is that this type of respect will be a lot more limiting.

What I have come to realize is that respect and gratitude hold similar spaces for us. They are both mindsets that reflect in our actions. If you can appreciate something or someone, you are more likely to act in a way that shows respect. If you respect someone or an idea, then you are more likely to show appreciation or have gratitude.

So why are gratitude and respect important for teens? Research into gratitude shows that it increases quality of life and overall health and happiness for teens and adults. New research from neuroscience supports gratitude as a natural antidepressant. Research into respect — and I don't mean just respecting adults — shows the same results. It's clear that gratitude and respect form the basis of a mindset that can help teens navigate the challenges that arise.

Because in my work with teens gratitude and respect are cut from the same cloth, I will discuss them together throughout the rest of this chapter. I share below themes as they relate to gratitude and respect from my work with teens.

Respect For Everything

Conversations about teens not having respect usually center around how teens treat or really respond to adults and mostly to adult requests. While this is a part of respect, respect is so much more. It's really about respect for everyone and everything.

I have come across the idea that we do not have to respect people's beliefs, only their right to have them. I would say there's a sweet spot in the middle. Of course we don't have to and most of us don't want to respect the beliefs of hate groups, criminal elements or those who are just looking to do harm; that being said, we can respect different beliefs that aren't extreme positions without agreeing.

Respect does flow to everything — even to inanimate objects. Try not to have me committed before I explain. This is not worship of inanimate objects like cars or clothes and it's not even assigning monetary value; it's about respect in the way we use, treat and care for them. Respect certainly applies to anything living. When it comes to other humans, we at least need to start with the premise that every human being deserves respect to the degree that we can give it. The same can be said for and applied to all other life.

Teens can adopt this notion of respect for everything. They do well when they do. We know that at times it isn't always easy. Teens want to throw that coat on the floor or fail to pick up trash when they're in a hurry. Having respect for all life and everything around them helps teens feel a sense of satisfaction. This mindset also helps teens to gain the respect of others.

Gratitude Is About Little Things

We all can appreciate big things and I would say most of us do. In some ways, teens are wired to appreciate the little things more than the big things. In part, this is due to where they are at developmentally and also their life experience. This is why they can get really excited about seeing a friend or getting a text from them, regardless of the content. I will say though that somewhere along the way they lose this. It's almost as if they think being an adult means not having gratitude for the little things. Sometimes teens get stressed out or overwhelmed by what they think they have to have or accomplish, so the little things start to become trivial. Adults can help in this regard by showing teens that this isn't true.

Appreciation and feeling grateful for the little things actually helps teens appreciate the bigger things even more. I feel strongly that life is made up of a lot of little things with a few big ones thrown in along the way. If we don't appreciate or have gratitude for the little things, life will be tougher than it has to be. Noticing all the little things can help teens appreciate what they do have even in bad situations.

We live in a society that tells us how bad we are if don't have the best of everything, and with much marketing geared towards teens, it's not a surprise that gratitude for what they have slowly fades. We know gratitude is woven together with respect, and when teens are able to appreciate the little things, respect becomes more attainable.

Perspective

Respect and gratitude continue to develop as teens move further along in their own development. This continued development is important for teens in developing perspective or perspective taking. In what is referred to as 'the developed world', we take many things for granted. Many of us have never and will never know what it's like to go hungry or not have clean water or to worry that our houses or neighborhoods will be under attack. We won't know extreme poverty or have to feel an oppressive regime. Teens are a reflection of our society. The perspective they have is due in large part to what they are exposed to. If they see an adult society that takes things for granted as a matter of course and is a behavior that is celebrated, they adopt this perspective as well.

As teens develop perspective, they are able to see issues from many angles. It improves their relationships with peers and adults. Imagine a teen being able to see your point of view. This comes from developing respect and gratitude and the perspective that comes along with that. To be clear, I am not suggesting that because those of us in the developed world are used to certain luxuries we aren't capable of gratitude or respect. It's just that we tend to overlook our good fortune, especially when it comes to meeting our basic needs. Because our basic needs are met, we move on and focus on other things. Perspective is key. We can go further and say that perspective is a necessary ingredient of gratitude and respect.

Teens need perspective, especially in today's world where we are so connected and the issues of the day demand gratitude and respect in order to resolve them equitable and sustainably.

So What Do We Do Now?

Our society's what-have-you-done-for-me-lately ideology manifests in a variety of ways. One is the lack of time to appreciate little things or to come from a place of gratitude. In addition, just uttering these words can get you sideways looks, or for some gives license for them to think of you as simple, unmotivated and out of touch with reality. Teens pick up on these thoughts.

Life, for sure, has its moments and what I am talking about here is not the idea of sunshine and rainbows all the time. There are times when respect and gratitude are stretches for all of us and teens are no exception. What I will say is that spending some time and energy on teens having more of this in their lives is worth it. Gratitude and respect, simply put, are important parts of teen health and happiness. They both have the power to change every aspect of a teen's life.

The changes will look different for each teen. I have witnessed changes from positive shifts in relationships to newfound motivation based on understanding. Teens respond well to having more gratitude and respect in their lives. It usually doesn't take much for teens to start seeing and feeling the changes. Once they do, they continue to see the value in continuing to bring this into their lives. Even though they will stumble sometimes, the trick is to keep going forward.

There are some simple ways to increase gratitude and respect in teens' lives, which I will share in the examples and recommendations section. Throughout this book we have been using questions at the end of each chapter to help with reflection. Below are some questions to help with that process.

Of course, you do not have to use any of the questions. These questions are not about a right or wrong answer. Don't worry about what you think the answers are supposed to be; just answer as honestly as you can. These questions are designed to get you to reflect and think about gratitude and respect. You may find that just answering these questions provides new insight or a new perspective. So whether you're a teen or adult reading this book, the questions are here to get you to think about learning.

As with all the questions in this book, grab a piece of paper and a pen, get comfortable, sit back, relax and have fun answering the following questions:

- *Question 1:* Who is/are the particular person/people or group of people that the teen/s in your life admires/admire?
- *Question 2:* What are the ideas or beliefs that the teen/s in your life seem to admire?

- *Question 3:* Describe the teen/s in your life's actions when it comes to gratitude.
- *Question 4:* Describe what you think the teen/s in your life feels/feel about the idea of respect for everyone and everything?
- *Question 5:* What are discussions and interactions like with the teen/s in your life when it comes to gratitude and respect?

As with all the questions in this book, I suggest revisiting these questions from time to time to note any changes and to see your progress. These questions are a guide to exploration and I invite you to come up with your own.

The following recommendations and examples are taken directly from the thoughts shared with me by teens and my own observations and practices. Just like with all the recommendations and examples in this book, they are not meant to be comprehensive. They are the major, relevant themes that have come from my work.

Recommendations/Examples

Respect Must Be Mutual

I remember sitting at a board meeting with about a dozen other adults. We were talking about the idea of respectful integrations between adults and teenagers. One board member spoke and while positioning is right hand above his head said, "Adults up here," and keeping his right had where it was, he positioned his left hand at his waistline and said, "Kids down here." If you adhere to that same philosophy, then the rest of this section probably isn't for you. Plus, you most likely find yourself having difficult relationships with teenagers or any child.

You can't expect a teen to respect you if you aren't giving respect to them. Some adults feel that teens should automatically respect them because they are adults. They should respect you because you're a human and they should start any interaction with you from a place of respect. You, as an adult, would want to do the same.

Respect is crucial for teens. It's something that they crave. And this does have to do with where they are developmentally. They are in the stage were they can formulate complex ideas and ways to solve problems. Keep in mind that some of them are quickly approaching, are at or just above the legal age of adulthood. In reality, teens want what any of us want and that is to be treated with respect and treated fairly. Unquestionably, adults have more life experience, and in general, the decisions they make have higher stakes attached to them. Sometimes that gets confused with the need for mutual respect, the thinking is that adult status automatically entitles us to more respect.

One of the most common themes I hear from teens is about this very idea. Tiffany, who had just turned 17, recently shared her thoughts with me on this very idea. "You know, some adults think that they should treat us like we are less than they are. I don't think that's right; really, it's disrespectful. It's hard for me to respect an adult who I know doesn't respect me. You know, I get that adults are more experienced than me and I respect adults or I think I do. I can tell when an adult respects me and it makes me feel like I can trust them. When they don't respect me, I probably won't even listen to what they have to say."

I have spoken with adults who think that mutual respect is about turning over full power to teens, as if they will not have any at all. Mutual respect isn't about giving away your right to respect. It's about sharing respect. There is one simple way to do this above all else and that is to take teens seriously and to give their thoughts, beliefs and feelings real consideration. Let them make decisions. Even when you don't agree with them, be honest about why you don't. Treat teens the way you want to and expect to be treated.

Remember, respect is critical for teens, so if you want to be a part of teens' lives and contribute to their health and happiness, please do all that you can to live the idea of mutual respect.

Practice Gratitude

Gratitude needs to be nurtured and attended to. It's not enough to just have a mindset of gratitude. A practice of gratitude shouldn't be a chore. It's about cultivating appreciation and understanding. A practice of gratitude also doesn't have to be complicated.

Practicing gratitude with teens is a lot like any other practice. First, you have to make time and space for it. One of the practices I like to do with teens is to set aside time for a gratitude session or gratitude. It really doesn't matter what you call it, it's all about setting aside time for appreciation. The appreciation can be for people or really anything. It's just about the practice of recognizing that there are things to be grateful for. I never made it formal or had rules. It was just a time for recognition.

Some of my friends and colleagues have worked with teens on making gratitude lists. The lists were not shared for the most part. If they were, I know that they only did this once trusting relationships were established. The idea is for teens to focus on things that they do have rather than what they don't. Another helpful part of a gratitude practice is to have gratitude even in the face of challenges. Teens will see the value in appreciation of the little things, challenges and what they already have. As adults, we can be helpful if we adopt these practices ourselves. A gratitude practice takes nurturing and attention. In the end, it's worth it. I have seen gratitude practice work well for teens and have a positive impact and even change their outlook.

Rene, who finished her first year of college, explained how a gratitude practice helped her through some challenging times. "I wonder where I would be if I didn't practice gratitude. It wasn't hard; I made it pretty simple. I would just take some time each day to think about someone I appreciated. It could be for something they helped me with or just who they were. Sometimes I thought about something that happened that I appreciated. I even thought about things, like, that I had food and clothes. There were a lot of little things too like my favorite song. This helped me through times where I felt lost, when I was overwhelmed or when things felt like they were going all wrong."

The practice of gratitude is an important part of teen health and happiness. Please consider working through it with the teens in your life.

Actions

We all strive to live what we believe or 'practice what we preach'. When it comes to respect, our actions do speak volumes. There will be times when we and the teens in our lives will act in a way that is counter to respect.

180

There are a variety of reasons as to why this happens, and even though we don't know exactly why it happens, we know that it does. Teens understand this struggle and they know it isn't easy. They also know that actions are important. As with many of the recommendations in this book, adults can be helpful by providing an example for teens. Adults can also help teens process actions that are respectful and ones that aren't.

"I always wondered if respect was one of those 'I'll-know-it-when-I-see-it' deals." This was what one parent put out to a group of adults and teens at a gathering in a local meetinghouse. As we talked through it and dove deep into what respect looks like in action, the following thoughts were shared.

We all acknowledged that when you have respect for everyone and everything, there are many ways that this shows up. It can even be a small act of kindness that a teen does because they have respect for that person. Actions that show respect are always about acting in a positive way towards a person or thing. It can be a positive word or picking up a piece of trash.

When all is said and done, it's about how we treat each other. Respect is contagious and so is disrespect. This is strikingly true with teens and even more so when teens witness adults being either respectful or disrespectful. It's like a road map for teens; it gives them something to steer by. It's true that teens can be either respectful or disrespectful all on their own and they do bear responsibility.

This is one of my favorite quotes from a teen on respectful action: "I think people notice when you are trying to act in a respectful way. Even though they might make fun of you for it, deep down they admire it. It doesn't have to be a big thing; it could be helping someone get through a door. But the big things matter too, because I think people notice the big things and notice when you aren't even trying to act in a respectful way."

As adults, we can have real conversations about respect with teens and what respectful actions look like. We can practice them and ask teens to practice them. At the end of the day, we all want to feel respected and have others around us feel respected.

Chapter Twelve

Get Outside/Play

In other sections of this book I have touched on the importance of getting outdoors and the transformative power of nature. In our current political climate, it seems that if you spend time outdoors, you are labeled by the way you spend that time outdoors: If you spend time outdoors hiking and exploring or working towards conservation, you are a left-wing socialist, head-in-the-clouds hippie; if you spend time outdoors hunting and fishing or raising animals, you are a right-wing conservative, mean-spirited buffoon.

Equally important and equally overlooked is the value of play. In much the same way as spending time outdoors, the idea of play in our culture has somehow been co-opted. It used to be synonymous with relaxation and joy and now it has come to mean frivolity, laziness and avoidance.

It's interesting to me that teens have a natural inclination towards play, but as they get further into their teen years, they come to believe that leaving play behind makes them more of an adult. Indeed, play evolves and as we develop, we tend to move to other areas of interest and types of play. Playing isn't just for kids. In fact, play is just as important for adults and teens. I have chosen to not separate these two ideas since I feel that they are closely related. Certainly, we can play without being outside and we can be outside without playing, at least in the conventional sense. Conservative estimates suggest that teens today spend about half as much time outside than they did even a decade ago.

The myriad benefits to physical health of spending time outdoors are many. Recently, there have been studies conducted on the mental health benefits of spending time outdoors. Some of those benefits include clearing your mind, increased focus, increased creativity, feeling good about yourself and an overall sense of well-being or stress reduction and happiness. Spending time outside has been shown to help people heal faster, whether that be mentally, physically or spiritually. Spending time outdoors has also been shown to kick your brain into high gear; the effects can be greater than caffeine. Interestingly and not coincidentally, the benefits of play are similar.

Before moving on, I would like to make a distinction between unstructured and unsupervised play and the structured, oversupervised variety. While there is benefit to structured and supervised play, as Peter Gray writes so eloquently about, there is greater benefit in the unstructured/unsupervised variety. In this chapter, the focus will be on the latter. As teens progress through their teen years, the type of play they tend to engage in is the more structured variety that is governed by rules and outcomes. What I see is that teens need more of the impromptu, spontaneous type of play that doesn't have hard-and-fast rules or outcomes.

I share below the thoughts from teens as it relates to being outdoors and play, as well as the results of my work.

Get Outside

The idea of being outdoors often conjures up images of an outdoor sport like rock climbing, skiing, whitewater rafting and a variety of others. While these are great ways to spend time outdoors, the reality is that just spending time in the outdoors has benefit. I find that being outside and doing nothing has great benefit. In fact, it is something I have recommended to most every teen I have worked with and will most likely continue to do so.

184

I always suggest finding a green and as quiet and secluded place as possible. Many think that getting outside would be a relatively easy thing for teens to do. I am here to tell you that for most teens this isn't easy. With the overscheduled existence, most teens have little time for it. Somehow the attraction of being indoors has become greater, and yes, technology has a role in that, as well as media in all its forms. Teens are naturally driven towards the various forms of media, and with so much at their fingertips, it's no wonder being indoors seems so fun.

Think about TV media; depending on what teens have access to, they can have thousands of a variety of shows to choose from. With services such as Netflix, Hulu and Amazon Prime, there are even more that can be accessed at any time and can be 'binge watched'. Teens also feel the pressure of our culture to constantly appear productive or engaged in anything deemed productive and just being outside is usually not one of those things.

The benefits of just being outside are real. I am reminded of Jalen, who came to me feeling, in his words, "stressed, frazzled and overwhelmed." Among other things, I asked him to try sitting and doing nothing outside, starting with five minutes a day. Within two weeks, he reported feeling more calm and less overwhelmed and increased the amount of time doing this to ten minutes or more.

So it isn't always about having to be active or doing something outdoors; it's just about being out there, realizing that, in part, this helps with reflection and allows thoughts and feelings to catch up, along with the many other benefits.

Play As A Priority

It is natural for humans to want to play. What's more is that we need it. Teens most definitely need it, but it has become less of a priority. If we view play as spontaneous activity engaged in for the purpose of joy and/or recreation where imagination and creativity can flourish, we can see the real need for play in teens' lives.

Looking at this from another angle, if play helps to increase and relate creativity and if creativity is something that today's employers value, there is a practical aspect to play. As Peter Gray suggests, play is how humans have learned for centuries. Kids used to mimic adults through play, and therefore, learn the necessary skills and norms to be well-adjusted contributing adults.

Play has also been shown to increase positive emotions, have a positive impact on relationships and an overall engagement with life. So play may not be so frivolous after all. Play is critical to healthy teen development and self-exploration. In my own work, I have watched as play has dwindled or increased in the life of a teen and the difference is noticeable and drastic at times. If I could say only one thing about play, I would say that as a priority it should not take a back seat to anything, unless it be a matter of survival.

I would add that play can be as easily made a priority as anything else we choose to prioritize. At the very least, we shouldn't shut it down. I have heard concerns from adults that somehow if teens are allowed to break into spontaneous play whenever and wherever the mood strikes them, they will develop the idea that life is all about play. Teens have better discretion than that. They know that there is a time and place for play. Yes, teens are impulsive at times and they are also observant and able to understand that life isn't only about play but that play can be about life.

If we are serious about helping teens be happier and healthier, then play must take its proper place as a top priority, for without it, teens will be devoid of spontaneity, joy, creative outlets and innovation.

Nature As A Healer

You are likely familiar with the phrase 'the healing power of nature' or something similar. It's true, nature is a healer. My work with teens has taken me to therapeutic environments that used the healing power of nature to help transform the lives of teens. Nature, the natural world, the outdoors all have this kind of power. I am not trying to make a claim that all one need do is to spend time in nature and all will be healed. The therapeutic environments I was part of used the healing power of nature along with other methods. I have been witness to major shifts in teens' health and happiness when the healing power of nature was embraced. There are whole fields in mental health called Nature Therapy or Eco-Therapy that are dedicated to using the natural world as a catalyst for healing and therapeutic breakthroughs.

In this section, I wrote about getting outside and some of the very real benefits of doing so. Viewing nature as a healer or embracing the healing power of nature is taking that idea further, recognizing that when a teen is struggling, perhaps there is an imbalance with their connection to the natural world. This imbalance happens all too easily for today's teens and it's all too easy to put the onus on them for this shortcoming.

As we have discussed, there are many factors at work here that are not always within the teen's control. There are many studies dating back decades that confirm the healing power of nature. A very famous one concluded that when hospital patients had a room with a view of nature, they healed more quickly than those that didn't. For teens, who, in most cases heal quicker than adults, nature can have an immediate impact. While this does take the idea of getting outside a little further because of the focus on the healing properties, this doesn't have to be complicated. It can be as simple as interacting with the natural world in some way, noticing its rhythms and cycles and the ability to heal itself over time.

We need to move away from the idea that we are somehow separate from the natural world, that the natural world is something to be shunned, conquered or feared and that if you value the natural world, you are tree hugger or are wasting your time. I have heard time in nature referred to as medicine for the soul and I would agree.

I end this section with one of my favorite quotes from Rachel Carson on the healing power of nature: "Those who contemplate the beauty of the earth find reserves of strength that will endure as long as life lasts. There is something infinitely healing in the repeated refrains of nature — the assurance that dawn comes after night and spring after winter."

So What Do We Do Now?

This is all great, but so what. What do we do now anyway? It's simple, as adults we can support the development and practical importance of play and time spent in the natural world. We can look to nature as being an aid and guide for healing or we can choose to ignore the myriad research that attests to the importance and need for both in the lives of teens. We don't want to force any of this on teens and the beauty of it is that in most cases we don't have to. The most we do is open a door or stand aside and let teens play and spend time outdoors.

In many places in this book, I have pointed to the hectic nature of many teens' schedules and the impact of such is perhaps even more noticeable when it comes to play and spending time outdoors, at least in the way they have been described here. I always suggest framing play as something that is enjoyed, spontaneous and as natural as breathing. Most environments are set up in antithesis to this idea and the message teens receive is that play is something that little kids do, and if you're truly mature, you don't play or at least your play is serious, competitive and purpose driven.

For far too many teens there is little time spent at play or in the outdoors where there isn't a scripted outcome or predetermined purpose. To say that this contributes to the pressure teens are under and to their health issues in various forms is a severe understatement.

In the recommendations and examples section, I share the reflections from teens that I have worked with over the years. I also add my own observations, where relevant.

As has been the case with most chapters, below are some questions to help with reflection. The questions are designed to help process the idea of play and getting outside.

Of course, you do not have to use any of the questions. These questions are not about a right or wrong answer. Don't worry about what you think the answers are supposed to be; just answer as honestly as you can. These questions are designed to get you to reflect and think about gratitude and respect. You may find that just answering these questions provides new insight or a new perspective.

So whether you're a teen or adult reading this book, the questions are here to get you to think about learning. As with all the questions in this book, grab a piece of paper and a pen, get comfortable, sit back, relax and have fun answering the following questions:

- *Question 1:* Describe your beliefs on play.
- *Question 2:* How does/do the teen/s in your life play?
- *Question 3:* How often does/do the teen/s in your life get outside?
- *Question 4:* How does/do the teen/s in your life spend his or her/their time outdoors?
- *Question 5:* What are the ways that the teen/s in your life can benefit from the healing power of nature?

As with all the questions in this book, I suggest revisiting these questions from time to time to note any changes and to see your progress. These questions are a guide to exploration and I invite you to come up with your own.

The following recommendations and examples are taken directly from the thoughts shared with me by teens and my own observations and practices. Just like with all the recommendations and examples in this book, they are not meant to be comprehensive. They are the major, relevant themes that have come from my work.

Recommendations/Examples

Find Or Create A Green Space

Connecting with the natural world can happen in many ways. One very real consideration is, what do teens who live in an urban setting or a setting that has little access to a natural setting do? For one, I have always been of the mind that we are part of the natural setting, not separate from it. We can find green spaces in urban settings. Having grown up in an area that did not have lots of green space or access to large open areas, I know that we can find green spaces if we seek them out. In the U.S., even the most densely populated urban areas have some amount of green space or have ones that you can access via public transportation. Central Park in Manhattan and Prospect Park in Brooklyn come immediately to mind. This may take more planning, but the results are well worth it.

Green spaces do pop up in unexpected places. While spending time in undisturbed natural spaces has increased benefits, we don't have to have soaring mountain ranges, fast-running rivers or endless miles of trails to enjoy and get the benefits of green spaces. Beaches, oceans and bodies of water do provide some of the same benefits; the effects though are a bit different than green spaces. Teens are pretty good at finding these places, especially with encouragement from adults. Adults can help by sharing some of their favorite green spaces with teens or by pointing out ones that they have come across.

When there is truly a lack of green space, teens can create their own. It could be as simple as doing some small plantings in a pot or clearing a space that would be green if it had a chance to grow. I have truly enjoyed working with teens in this capacity, helping them create a green space of their own — everything from community and rooftop gardens to cleaning up spaces in their community, and when possible, doing some plantings. It is such a rich experience and just like nature has healing power. Creating or helping to maintain green spaces has similar benefits that also come with learning, sense of accomplishment and enhancing the community.

Tara, who was part of a group of teens, had this to say: "When we were first talking about cleaning this area up and making a garden, I kinda laughed. I thought we weren't going to be able to do it and that the people in the neighborhood wouldn't allow it. We got started and then I wanted it to happen. I wanted it to look good and give me and other people a space to come to. It's true that I started to feel a little better than before we started. I guess I felt stressed a lot, but this helped with that."

It is possible and important for teens to find or create green spaces and spending even a short amount of time in them can be transformative.

Take A Hike

In contrast to creating green spaces, finding a place where teens can hike or walk in green spaces is important as well. I fully admit that there is an issue of access here; not every teen has immediate or reasonable access to places like this. I agree that it is a problem. What I can say is that there are programs that will help give teens, who would otherwise not have access to areas like this, access. Adults can help teens organize trips to places that do have access to walking among green spaces, like New York City's Central Park or Chicago's Lincoln Park. Of course, trips can be organized to more expansive green spaces that do not have to be expensive and can be done within a day.

In addition to the many benefits of hiking to teens' physical health, there are benefits to their mental health as well. Hiking has been shown to open up our minds and actually help us solve or move on from a problem. There have also been studies that show hiking can help to reduce the symptoms of ADHD in teens. One of the many things I love about hiking is that, for the most part, you do not need specialized training or skills. Depending where the teen is doing the hiking, there generally isn't specialized equipment needed as well. Most definitely, there are certain types of clothing and footwear that are recommended over others for hiking and it's always important to hydrate. While hiking safety is outside the scope of this book, there are many great websites like national and state parks or hiking organizations where you can find this information.

I have done a great deal of work with teens that had their first hiking experience ever. It is such a thrill to watch teens be opened up to a whole new world and activity that will have such a positive impact on their health and happiness. James, who had grown up in one of NYC's boroughs, said to me as we were taking a short break on the trail, "I will be coming back here hopefully a lot or I will find other places like this. This really feels good to me."

As adults, we can help teens by perhaps going with them or providing information to them. Adults can take the time to find out more about the benefits of hiking for teens to help them be able to take advantage of those benefits.

One of the biggest mistakes adults make is to want to interrupt and oversupervise play. As teens get older, this generally becomes a lesser issue; however, it does still occur. To be clear, if it's a safety issue, of course adults may need to interrupt or supervise. As adults, we need to resist our natural inclination to interrupt or oversupervise play in any way. Once we interrupt or try to intervene the natural process of play and creativity, the other benefits that come with it are diminished, if not lost entirely.

When teens have a chance to play in a way that is unhindered by adults, it is much more authentic and real. As I mentioned above, play is a way for teens to work out and learn about the adult world. If there are constructs placed on play or if it is interrupted so that adults can interject their ideas, is that really reflective of the adult world? And how joyful is that really?

I recall watching a group of teenagers who were playing some sort of game that I can only describe as a very humorous conglomeration of many different games. The teens were clearly having a ball and in my mind were being safe and inclusive. In fact, the game itself had no real physical contact or threat of injury. After about ten minutes, an adult, who seemed to be related in some way to at least one teen, came over to intervene. Almost immediately the joy was gone. When the teens picked the game back up, it was easy to see that it had shifted and they gave it up after about five more minutes. Sure, maybe they just got bored with it, but they didn't seem to be bored before the adult intervention.

The power of play is even more powerful when we are able to leave teens to their own devices, unless it is absolutely necessary to intervene. I

194

have heard over and over from teens how they wish adults would let them be during times like these.

Lloyd, a 16-year-old, told me one day how the adults in his life seemed to always feel the need in some way to supervise his play or intervene. He understood that if he were, say, playing video games all night that his parents would intervene on his behalf. What he didn't understand was why adults felt that their input was always necessary or sought after. "I know that adults are just trying to care about me. I don't always get why when I am doing something I enjoy or something that is like playing, they need to interrupt. Adults know more than me, but how do I learn on my own if they keep interrupting."

Chapter Thirteen

Sleep & Downtime

As a society, we are sleep deprived. The new norm is exhaustion. Exhaustion is somehow worn as a badge of honor; the more exhausted, worn out and tired you are and look, no matter the negative impact on your performance and health, the more points you earn. We have become too accustomed to bragging about how early we rise in the morning to go to work or how many hours we spend working with little regard to the impact on our health. Some of the latest polls show that over 40% of Americans get less than the recommended hours of sleep; some significantly so. This can have serious health consequences, as well as affecting our performance in work, school, recreational activities and in our relationships.

Sleep is when our body repairs, heals and rids itself of toxins. Sleep studies have shown that sleep is necessary for improved memory, physical and mental performance and creativity. Another benefit of sleep is that it reduces inflammation in our body, which is the root cause of many illnesses and diseases. Sleep is critical to overall health and happiness, yet most teens fall short of the recommended nine to nine-and-a-half hours of sleep per night. In general, as teens get older and busier, the amount of sleep they get decreases.

One of the main reasons for teen sleep deprivation, especially for teens that are in school, are school start times. Teens undergo a natural shift in their sleep patterns, which moves their natural time to fall asleep to around 11 pm or later. Add nine-and-a-half hours of recommended sleep to that time and we can see that most school start times are just too early for teens to function optimally.

196

Schools that have shifted to a later start time have seen improvements in everything from behavior and the ability to focus to quality of and enthusiasm for learning. As recommended in the chapter on learning, as important as a later start time is, many other factors should also be considered when choosing a learning environment.

Sleep deprivation has a number of effects on teen health and happiness. For one, it contributes to daytime sleepiness in teens. Other effects include, but are not limited to, irritability, weight gain, moodiness, inability to focus, hypertension, lethargy, difficulty waking up in the morning and brain fog. Sleep deprivation also makes it difficult for teens to ever know what it's like to feel good, as they get used to going through life feeling tired or in a daze.

It is clear that sleep is a vital part of teen health and happiness and we know that teens don't get enough of it for a variety of reasons. We have to figure out a way to hit the sweet spot between teens being active and engaged to sleep-deprived zombie teens that are putting their health and happiness at risk.

Perhaps equally important as sleep is the need for teens to have downtime. I mean just that, downtime; not sitting and doing a predetermined task, but actual downtime. Downtime gives teens a much-needed mental break and also allows time for quiet reflection. The Italians have a saying, "Be la bellezza del far niente" or "Il dolce far niente," which means, 'the beauty of doing nothing'. In my work, I have noticed how difficult this can be for some teens, especially with all the electronic distractions our society now has at the constant ready. I have also witnessed how even a few minutes a day of this can make a difference.

Some of my colleagues suggest that if teens are doing something during downtime that they enjoy and is not imposed, like a playing a video game, journaling or texting, that this has the same benefits. I say it depends on the activity. Downtime away from electronic stimulation has been shown to decrease stress, quiet the mind and lead to better sleep quality. I am a big proponent of downtime. With the many pressures that teens are under today, they don't get nearly enough of it.

One of the most common complaints I hear from teens is that they feel overscheduled. With all the activities they try to cram into a day along with the demands of school, and for some part-time jobs, it's little wonder that teens feel they have little downtime or 'time to themselves'. Lack of downtime may seem trivial or be put into the 'get-over-it, no-one-gets-enough-downtime' category. While the latter may be true, it still doesn't make it a good thing. When teens don't get enough downtime, they have higher rates of depression, illness related to stress, increased instances of suicidal thoughts and have more emotional and mental health issues.

Downtime helps teens get to know themselves; without it, they don't get the time they need to let their thoughts play out or to reflect on and think through the situations they are confronted with every day. This shouldn't be confused with obsessive rumination or overthinking to the point where it causes unnecessary angst, fear or inaction.

It's evident that sleep and downtime are vital aspects of teen health and happiness. It's also evident that most teens are not getting enough of either for the reasons alluded to in this chapter and others. This chapter goes right into the recommendations for sleep and downtime, as they will give enough frame to understand their aspects. The following recommendations are from my work with teens and my own observations on sleep and downtime.

So What Do We Do Now?

Our culture has become obsessed with the idea that in order to contribute meaningfully to society, you have to be exhausted to a notch above death. The idea goes further to include any downtime or idle time as a folly, kids stuff or a waste of time, or worse, used as fodder to further fuel the lazy teen caricature. We have gotten to the point where routines, such as school start times or packing days full of activities, if they are ever questioned, are only done so in the abstract. Little, if any, action is taken to change these 'norms' that we have become accustomed to for a variety of legitimate reasons.

Caught up in all this are teenagers — most of whom have lives that include overscheduled days, weeks, months and years, to the point where they aren't comfortable when every minute isn't scheduled. In turn, this has an impact on their health and happiness, since in order to fit everything in, they are sleep deprived and are lacking in any real downtime or time to themselves that doesn't have some sort of outcome attached to it. It would be hard to find many who think that teens shouldn't have access to a variety of activities. I agree that all teens should have access to a variety of activities that they enjoy and can find meaning in. At the same time, teens needn't have every moment of their lives taken up with one or multiple activities.

In the chapter on passion, we discussed its importance and that when teens find one or more passions, they will likely spend a lot of time doing them. Stories abound of the sports hero, musician or Olympian who spent countless hours as a teen practicing and competing. What gets lost in that context is that sleep and downtime were important factors, especially for the athletes. In fact, most professional athletes will tell you how important sleep is to optimal performance and recovery.

Below are recommendations and suggestions to best support sleep and downtime based on my time spent with teens and my own observations. Like we have been doing throughout this book, we will start with questions to help with reflection. In the event that you aren't reading this book chapter by chapter, I have been providing some suggestions about how to approach answering these questions.

Of course, you do not have to use any of them. These questions are not about a right or wrong answer. Don't worry about what you think the answers are supposed to be; just answer as honestly as you can. It's about bringing awareness to what is happening and having time for reflection. You may find that just answering these questions provides new insight or a new perspective.

So whether you're a teen or adult reading this book, the questions are here to get you to think about sleep and downtime and their importance to teen health and happiness. If you're an adult that isn't a parent to teens but works with teens, answer the questions based on what you have observed from working with teens.

As with all the questions in this book, grab a piece of paper and a pen, get comfortable, sit back, relax and have fun answering the following questions:

- *Question 1:* Based on the recommended amount of hours of sleep for teens, would you say the teen/s in your life is/are getting enough sleep? Why did you answer the way you did?

- *Question 2:* Do you discuss the importance of sleep with the teen/s in your life?

- *Question 3:* Are there any changes that can be made so that the teen/s in your life can get enough sleep?

- *Question 4:* Does/do the teen/s in your life have enough unscheduled downtime with no outcomes attached?

- *Question 5:* What are the challenges to the teen/s in your life getting enough downtime? What has to change so that they do?

As with all the questions in this book, I suggest revisiting these questions from time to time to note any changes and to see your progress. These questions are a guide to exploration and I invite you to come up with your own.

Recommendations/Examples

Help Create Good Conditions For Sleep

Adults who work with teens but don't have teens of their own may think that this is outside of their control. Of course you cannot create the physical conditions; what you can help create is the space for exploring the importance of sleep and the study of sleep science. If you work with teens in a capacity that requires them to come to you, you can create schedules that include reasonable start and finish times and duration of time spent together.

201

You can also ensure that any related task you give them that they have to do outside of their time spent with you is realistic and will not require an inordinate amount of time that will deprive them of sleep — at the very least, not consistently.

The optimal physical conditions for sleep are a room that is devoid of noise and light, to the degree that is possible. This has been one of the easiest fixes to ensure the best sleep for teens.

Christina, who was starting her 11th grade year, told me about how she had a hard time sleeping at night and how most days she woke up not feeling refreshed. As we talked through the physical conditions she was in during sleep, we found that there was too much light getting into the room and that she had pets in her room that would make noise in their enclosures at night. When she was able to cut down on the light coming in and placed the pets in another room, the quality of her sleep improved.

Temperature of the room is also important. According to Arianna Huffington's new book, "The Sleep Revolution," the optimal room temperature to promote the best sleep is 67 degrees Fahrenheit. This may seem overly chilly to some, but being overheated does not promote good sleep. I also recommend encouraging teens to turn off or remove as many electronic devices as possible from their rooms and to stop screen time about 30 minutes before bed.

Make Sleep Important

Rather than tell teens to suck it up if they don't get enough sleep, we need to help make sleep important in their lives. Most adults do not have actual control over the sleeping habits of teens. As many parents can attest, even when teens are in their beds, they can be up to the wee hours doing various things. I firmly believe that portable and stationary electronic devices have increased this phenomenon. Many teens report texting their friends or playing video games into the early morning hours, in part due to access to these devices, their overscheduled days and the natural rhythms of teen brains.

We have to make sure we don't leave sleep as the last thing on the list when it comes to health and happiness. We can provide resources to teens so that they can understand the importance of sleep. As adults, we can also be understanding when teens are sleep deprived. If we notice that it is interfering with their health and happiness, we can notify the proper adults, when appropriate, so that they may intervene on teens' behalf.

Sleep isn't something we should leave to chance or expect that it will take its rightful place as a foundation of teen health and happiness if we don't recognize its importance. Teens may not always be responsive to this idea, but they will respect it if it comes from the right place. If it appears to be just another adult tactic to control their lives and keep them from having fun, then the likelihood of teens being receptive is not very high.

I remember talking to Paul, who was in his 12th grade year, about the importance of sleep. "I never thought sleep was that important. I thought it was more for, like, younger kids. I did start to notice that when I didn't get enough sleep, I didn't always feel great. When I read that athletes make sure they get good sleep, I knew it was good for me too."

Simply put, as adults we have to be conscious of the need for teens to have downtime. Cramming as many activities or tasks into their days as possible creates a host of issues, some of which have been discussed in this chapter. We must help teens create time in their days for downtime. One of the best ways to do that is not to fall into the trap of exalting exhaustion and overwork because we want them to have good work habits and ethics. Another way we can do this is to actually talk with teens about downtime and what that might look like for them. Placing value on it doesn't ensure that teens will engage in it, though it does give it a space in their consciousness.

In the same way that we can help create good conditions for sleep, we can create good conditions for teens to have downtime. Being mindful of their schedules, what they need to complete (other than what we may ask of them) and providing downtime when they are with us, if that is possible. One of techniques I've used in pretty much any of my time spent with teens is to make time for downtime. For the most part, these were not long stretches of time, as even a few minutes is helpful.

I recommend at least an hour per day of downtime. I've received many eye-rolls over the years when proposing this. All I can say is that ensuring that teens have this downtime has helped teens that I have worked with to feel more at ease, focused and in touch with what is going on around them.

Above I mentioned a few of the health challenges not getting enough downtime poses for teens. Teens today feel enormous pressure, and contrary to popular wisdom, they do actually do a lot, aren't lazy, are involved in many things and have real-life pressures. Making time for downtime is the least we can do for teens. I can tell you that even if they don't take you up on it, they will very much appreciate the fact that you are supportive of their need for it. In a real way, providing them with downtime shows them that it's okay to be comfortable with downtime.

A teen I worked with named Tracy comes to mind. At 15, she seemed years older, and when I listened to her talk about her schedule and her belief that any idle time was wasted time, she sounded more like an older adult to me than a teenager. Of course, I didn't want to stop her from engaging in the things that she enjoyed, though we did find out she didn't always enjoy all of them. What I set out to do was to have her discover the importance of downtime and how I could help her create it.

It was difficult at first, because she had been so conditioned over the years that downtime became uncomfortable for her. I made time for downtime during our meetings. Eventually, she was able to do so for herself and it became something that she valued more than she did prior to our work together. I don't think it ever really became first on her list of priorities, but I believe it was in the top ten, where before it wasn't even on the list.

"This wasn't easy for me, you know. I never had really made time for it. I didn't think it was a good thing. I enjoy it now, but I don't think I got up to an hour yet." What I noticed after we did this for a bit is that she seemed more focused, more clear-headed, she was able to stay on a thought longer and I would say she became more aware of herself.

Chapter Fourteen

Bringing It All Together

A lot has been discussed in the previous chapters and this chapter is about tying them together in a way that will help adults support teens in the challenges they face to their health and happiness. Teens do face a myriad of challenges when it comes to their health and happiness, from millions of dollars on advertising that specifically targets them, to a lack of access to truly healthy options, to continuous pressure from an adult society that values things more than health and common misconceptions adults harbor with regard to teens.

Below are the top three misconceptions I have come across that adults have about teens when it comes to health and happiness.

Misconception One: Teens Don't Care About Their Health

This is perhaps the most damaging of all the misconceptions. Sure, we can probably all remember when we were young and point to examples of today's teens indulging in eating 'junk food' and some other not-so-healthy behaviors. This, however, does not mean teens do not care about their health. In fact, many teens use the Internet and media to research health topics, especially those that are important to them, such as reproductive and sexual health. What tends to happen is that adults want teens to care about the health topics they feel are important. As well meaning as this is, teens will not always feel the same way.

When teens don't change their behavior or understand why they should or how they could, adults often take this as a sign that they don't care about their health. This is not the case; teens care a great deal about their health when it makes sense to them.

Misconception Two: Teens Don't Want To Change

Change is perhaps one of the most difficult of all life's challenges for any group of people. We all get set in our ways and our routines. This is not always a detriment to health, as healthy routines have a positive effect on our health.

Teens, like any group of people, are probably going to be a bit resistant to change at first. In my experience, teens can be a lot more flexible when it comes to change, and once they have a chance to try out the change, they take to it more readily and sustainably than adults. The change needs to make sense to them. They need to know why they are doing it, how it is going to help them now and how to implement the change in a way that best lines up within their life. Teens will make changes when they know how, why and when it makes sense within their lives.

Misconception Three: Teens Are Lazy

I can't tell you how often I hear adults lament about how lazy 'today's teens' are and how, even when they know what they should be doing and how to do it, they won't do it because they are too lazy; yet millions of teens are involved in organized sports, millions in after-school activities and millions in summer camps. Of course, statistics alone do not tell the whole story, but this at least gives some insight into what teens are up to and to the fact that they aren't lazy. We don't need statistics to tell us that teens' days are often highly scheduled, running from one activity to another. Teens are not lazy, and if there is any shred of teen laziness, perhaps we need to examine our adult culture and how sedentary in mind, body and spirit some adults have become.

If we can address these misconceptions honestly, it will go a long way in helping teens empower themselves so that they can take charge of their health and happiness. It is difficult to feel empowered when misconceptions abound to the point where they create barriers for teens taking action for their health and happiness.

I have received the following criticisms over the years, or perhaps more accurately, accusations that I paint a far too rosy picture of teens, dismissing any of the mistakes and bad choices they make. I suppose that there may be some truth in that; however, I think it would be more accurate to say that I don't focus on them. What I focus on is helping teens learn from them or to avoid them altogether by learning about themselves and what they need.

Below are some highlights that I believe capture the spirit of this book.

Use What You Can

At the beginning of this book, I suggested that you may come across some things that you don't agree with, seemed hokey or impractical or were counter to your own experience. I also suggested that you discard what you think isn't useful or put it aside for another time. In the same way that adults reading this book may do this, so too will teens. I ask that any adult reading this book allow teens to do this for themselves with guidance.

Take away from this book what you feel is immediately relevant based on the needs of the teen and try it out. If it works, keep on that path. Start slow. It would be difficult to implement all of these suggestions at once, plus I don't recommend it.

Some experts in the field recommend changing every aspect of a teen's life at once, suggesting that it is the only way to true transformation. My thoughts on this are twofold. One is that in the most extreme circumstances this can work, as I have witnessed and been involved in its success. However, this truly should be reserved for the most extreme circumstances and only under the strict guidance of medical professionals, as there are many factors involved, including teen resistance. The flip side is that doing this may very well cause teens much additional stress and anxiety and the feeling of being out of control. Remember, this is also about collaborating with teens on these suggestions in a way that is realistic and doable.

Be Open, Be Flexible

As has been mentioned, some of what you read in this book may seem out there. I understand. I still come across ideas that just don't seem to add up at the moment. What I have included in this book are the aspects that have worked for improving teen health and happiness. I also have included my observations and the reflections and ideas of teens on what has worked for them.

You may find that trying a suggestion from this book doesn't seem to be working or perhaps is working in a different way than expected. This is when it is important to be flexible, knowing that the suggestions in this book are not hard-and-fast rules. In collaboration with teens, modify and adapt the suggestions to fit the unique context, when necessary.

In our current society, we are overloaded with information and claims that seem too good to be true. There are certainly those out there that are selling 'snake oil', so it only follows that we are skeptical and I think we should be. I remain cautious but open to ideas and suggestions when it comes to integrating best practices for teen health and happiness. If we can do this as adults, we then can support teens as they learn what will be best for their health and happiness.

The example of acupuncture comes to mind. Turn back the clock to twenty or even thirty years ago when acupuncture was not common in Western medicine, especially in the U.S. Now some insurance companies will cover acupuncture treatments and some medical professionals recommend acupuncture as a course of treatment. I, myself, went to a center that included a Western MD/ neurologist, an acupuncturist and Tuina massage therapist. I bring this up to illustrate how remaining open to suggestions and ideas can bring about positive changes to teen health and happiness.

Keep Exploring And Learning

We live in the age of research and there does seem to be something new uncovered or proven, to the degree that it can be, every day. I always recommend continued learning and exploration right alongside teens.

As you read through the chapters of this book and looked at what was included with relation to the aspects and recommendations, you may have thought, what about this, what about that, why wasn't this included? Again, this is a reflection of my experiences and the experiences of the teens I have been so fortunate work with. Undoubtedly, this book has limitations, which is why it is critical that adults and teens keep learning and exploring together.

There are so many fields of knowledge to draw from, including that of your own experience and the experience of the teens in your life. There are a lot of people doing good work in the name of teen health and happiness, which is knowledge you can draw from as well.

Give Yourself & Teens A Break

Discussing areas of this book with adults, common thoughts that were expressed were a variation of this: I must be or I feel like a crappy parent/teacher/coach/counselor and the list goes on. While there exists an extremely small percentage of adults who dislike teens and go out of their way to make the life of teens difficult, the overwhelming majority of adults do not fall into this category. I am not in the habit of making guarantees, but I will bet that most adults really do want what is best for teens and want them to be healthy and happy.

Adults, you have to give yourself a break. You're doing the best that you can. A slight reluctance I had in writing this book is that adults would read this book, toss it aside and say 'there is no way I can do all that' and come away feeling overwhelmed and perhaps even a little guilty. As fortunate as I am to have worked with and to continue to work with teens, I have had the same good fortune with adults. What I know from this work is

211

that adults expend a lot of effort and energy to do what is best for teens — at the very least, what they think is the best. So give yourself a break. The fact that you are reading this book should be an indication that you are willing to do what you can.

In the same spirit adults need to give teens a break, teens need to give adults and themselves a break. Being clear, this is about having realistic expectations, not the lack of expectations. I understand and have been swept up in it myself, the pressure that adults feel to help teens distinguish themselves in some way so they get into that great college, so that they can get that great job or be the next Michael Jordan or Sting. As we do this, we focus intensely on the next step, forgetting to enjoy and take away what we can from the here and now and from the process.

This pressure is hard on adults and it trickles down to the way they interact with teens. I know that many adults have felt that if teens would only listen or just do what they suggested, it would be so much easier on them. Teens are doing the best that they can. Yes, they are going to do things that seem counter to their health and happiness and they still want to be happy and healthy, as crazy as that might sound. If we can give ourselves and teens a break, recognizing that we all feel the various pressures of life and with that will come a whole lot of mistakes, missteps and ways of doing things that are out of balance, we can help teens empower themselves.

Final Thoughts

As we come to the end of this book, I share some final thoughts that I hope will bring all the aspects of this book together nicely.

Fundamentally, this book is about teens being empowered to take charge of their health and happiness with the guidance and support of adults. This only seems fitting, because in essence, we can't really empower anyone. We can just clear the way for them to empower themselves.

Teens have such great capacity for resiliency and complexity. Their health and happiness, to me, is a foundation not only of their success but of ours as well. We know that there are many aspects that make up an individual and that can impact their health and happiness. To look at health and happiness from only a physical lens or a spiritual lens is limiting.

Teen health and happiness is more than the sum of its parts and adult support is an intricate piece. I have witnessed such amazing transformations when teens and adults work together for teen health and happiness. We are in the midst of important times for our world and we need happy, healthy teens that are ready to engage with the world. If we can help teens empower themselves now, they will carry on these traits into adulthood. Health and happiness is freeing for both teens and adults.

This book has been a journey through my work with teens, whose lives I am so very lucky to have been a part of even for a short while. I focused on the positive outcomes and what worked for this book and that has come from understanding what also did not work. The only way that happened is by working with teens, being honest, open, flexible and authentic with a healthy side dish of humor.

I invite every teen and adult to do the same.

38156378R00125

Made in the USA
Middletown, DE
18 December 2016